CRYSTALS FOR HEALING

Crystals and Gemstones Have a Magical Healing Power

(Learn the Ultimate Techniques to Increase Your Spiritual Energy)

William Buckles

Published by Harry Barnes

William Buckles

All Rights Reserved

Crystals for Healing: Crystals and Gemstones Have a Magical Healing Power (Learn the Ultimate Techniques to Increase Your Spiritual Energy)

ISBN 978-1-7751430-7-9

All rights reserved. No part of this guide may be reproduced in any form without permission in writing from the publisher except in the case of brief quotations embodied in critical articles or reviews.

Legal & Disclaimer

The information contained in this book is not designed to replace or take the place of any form of medicine or professional medical advice. The information in this book has been provided for educational and entertainment purposes only.

The information contained in this book has been compiled from sources deemed reliable, and it is accurate to the best of the Author's knowledge; however, the Author cannot guarantee its accuracy and validity and cannot be held liable for any errors or omissions. Changes are periodically made to this book. You must consult your doctor or get professional medical advice before using any of the suggested remedies, techniques, or information in this book.

Upon using the information contained in this book, you agree to hold harmless the Author from and against any damages, costs, and expenses, including any legal fees potentially resulting from the application of any of the information provided by this guide. This disclaimer applies to any damages or injury caused by the use and application, whether directly or indirectly, of any advice or information presented, whether for breach of contract, tort, negligence, personal injury, criminal intent, or under any other cause of action.

You agree to accept all risks of using the information presented inside this book. You need to consult a professional medical practitioner in order to ensure you are both able and healthy enough to participate in this program.

Table of Contents

INTRODUCTION 1

CHAPTER 1: SO, WHAT ARE CRYSTALS? 3

CHAPTER 2: HERE ARE 8 USEFUL REMEDIES TO CURE YEAST INFECTION 39

CHAPTER 3: CRYSTALS AND CRYSTAL HEALING 67

CHAPTER 4: SELECTING YOUR CRYSTALS 74

CHAPTER 5: WHAT, EXACTLY, IS CHAKRA? 81

CHAPTER 6: THE POWER OF CRYSTAL 89

CHAPTER 7: THE USE OF CRYSTALS 109

CHAPTER 8: COLORS AND CHAKRAS 113

CHAPTER 9: CHOOSING THE RIGHT CRYSTAL 149

CHAPTER 10: WHAT IS CRYSTAL HEALING? 164

CHAPTER 11: STEPS TO MAKE AND ACTIVATE YOUR OWN CRYSTAL GRID 177

CHAPTER 12: POPULAR HEALING CRYSTALS FOR SPECIFIC PHYSICAL, EMOTIONAL, MENTAL AND SPIRITUAL NEEDS 185

CHAPTER 13: HOW TO CLEAN YOUR CRYSTAL 195

CHAPTER 14: GARNET 199

CONCLUSION 201

Introduction

Are you in for a great treat because you will be about to learn a new way of healing.

Being one of the species who were chosen to inhabit the Earth is a blessing for human kind because we live in an environment that has an abundant amount of resources which answer to any problem that we could possibly have. Everything that we need – from safety, security, up to daily provisions – is already provided for by nature. When it comes to healing, nature has also provided us with different natural ways on how to cure illnesses and ailments. We are well aware of herbal medicine and nature based alternative remedies that can heal our health problems as effectively as synthetic medicines but there is one way of healing that we are not yet so knowledgeable about. This natural way of healing is called crystal healing. If this is the first time that you have encountered this term or if you want to learn more about it, then you have certainly made a wise decision to buy this book because this is the best book for you to learn all about crystal healing.

In this book you will learn the basic information that will help you in becoming an expert in crystal healing. You will learn everything there is to know about this alternative way of curing such as its history and where it came from, how to heal using crystals and the different crystals that you can use in order to cure the common illnesses that people often experience.

Chapter 1: So, What Are Crystals?

The glowing of the crystal is like the emergence of new life. If one sees a crystal, one sees a picture of flowing colours. But what you are seeing is clusters of atoms and molecules that have established themselves. Crystal consists of different characteristics while offering many different sizes and shapes. People in today's world are adapting to new ways to heal themselves which might not always support scientific evidence, known as alternative medicine. And crystals have grasped the eyes of people, not recently, but since centuries. The properties of different crystals are considered to heal the body in different ways. To say it cleanly, it eliminates the negative energy flow of your body, while restoring your positive energy flow, also, preventing the entry of different types of diseases. The elements of the crystals determine how they are formed. If you want to see how crystals are formed, you can do a little experiment of yourself. It is completely safe. You just have to put a table salt available in your kitchen to your regular tap water. Leave it for 24 hours. What you will see after that time is the formation of many small, little crystal cubes. Here, the water is evaporating, bringing the atom of the salt to come closer with the tap water, its result making clusters of atoms that you can see from your naked eyes. Of course, the bond of all the crystals is formed that way: two atoms coming together. Some take a few days; some take the evolutionary approach: millions of years. Though the presence of crystals inside the earth is in a very small amount, they get made when the liquid inside the earth boils up at a tremendous temperature, and when the temperature cools down. These crystals are called natural crystals. In regards to this, nowadays, many crystals are formed inside the laboratory. Scientists can change the formations of crystals by changing their chemical compositions.

Crystals and their curative power

The popularity of crystals lies to its curative power by healing the body through vibration; you can call this a flow of energy. The history of using crystals is ancient; its practice dates back to 6,000 years. The people who use crystal believes that different crystals are filled with their healing power that relates to the mind, body, and soul. It is also said that crystals as medicine are borrowed from cultures belonging to Asia: Yin and yan, and Chi or Qi concepts in Chinese cultures. Also, crystals relate to the philosophies in Buddhism and Hinduism—the purification of chakras in a human body by using the different techniques that each crystal presents. The life-energies and its vortices, crystals possess such properties that the crystals tend to clear all the pathways, connecting all vortices, while allowing the radiant energy: life energy, to flow through your body. The key to achieving this at an exponential growth would require the acceptance of the current emotional state, mindfulness, and introspection; these combinations reflect the need for self-care. When one does that, along with using the different types of crystals, the growth in life possess a unique aura, giving individual various emotional benefits. There are many crystals available in the market, so before talking about their countless types, first, let's talk about the categories of crystals with their physical and chemical properties. They are metallic crystals, covalent crystals, Ionic crystals, and molecular crystals.

Metallic Crystals: They are made of metal elements. These crystals carry a lustrous sparkle with them while each metallic atom sits on the lattice sites, allowing the atoms to float freely around the lattice. Metallic crystals carry different properties. One of them is that they are very excellent conductors of heat and electricity. Think about our home, the electricity is provided by the copper wire that is extracted from the copper crystals.

Covalent crystals: The atoms in the covalent crystals carry pure covalent bonds between them. Whenever the atoms are shared in the electrons, this is where the covalent bonds exist. This bond is usually very strong and is hard to break. Think of diamonds, how adamantine they are. They of silicon carbide and quartz—they all are a pack of covalent bonds, which are very difficult to separate.

Ionic crystals: Here one atom which is negatively charged gets attracted to the atom that is positively charged. This phenomenon is known as electrostatic forces. Other names consist of charged bonds. Here the atoms are held together, usually arranged in a pattern based on the kind of charge each atom carries. The crystals that come out of the ionic bonds are usually solid and have a high melting point. Think about your table salt, or potassium chloride, or bromide.

Molecular crystals: They are formed from hydrogen bonds. They are usually considered as weak bonds as they usually contain recognizable molecules inside their structure. It is the non-covalent interactions. These crystals are soft because they contain hydrogen bonding.

Think of ice crystals, or the crystalline sugar, or dry ice.

From exterior to the atomic level, metaphysics guides us that crystals are geometrically perfect. Due to this perfect structure, the Dominant Oscillatory Rate of the crystal is very stable. But what is Dominant Oscillatory Rate you may ask? It is a vibrational frequency that our bodies carry. When the vibration is at a balanced state, the chance of achieving optimized health is very high, but there are many environmental factors that may allow the body to not be at a balanced state such as stresses, illnesses, and pollution. Even organs and all the body's cells have their own DOR. It is safe to say that our body's vibrational frequency can easily be disrupted when faced with environmental factors. But the good thing is that we can attune the vibrational frequency with the right source. Crystals provide a stable DOR. They even have their own healing properties that can help the individual to heal a particular problem. Although many complicated forms of crystal have their specific properties that heals a particular individual's ailment, but one thing is true for all the crystals: they possess within themselves a stable vibrational frequency. This simple knowledge can help you to differentiate the meaning of various crystals available in the market. As you are familiarized with its properties, so now let's discuss different crystals and what healing power they holds:

•**Jasper**: The ancient Egyptians associated the crystal Jesper with its help in the menstrual cycle of the women. The crystal helped the women during pregnancy and kept at bay spiders and scorpions during those times. Jasper crystals heal diseases relating to lungs, chest, and stomachs. Brown jasper crystals help to keep the toxins out of the body while strengthening the immune system. Yellow jaspers help the body to detoxify the emotions while restoring the digestive system in a calm state. The transformative power that the crystal jasper contains is that it provides you with the power to be honest with yourself when you are faced with difficulty. You assert the situation rather than showing aggression. Instead of being selfish, the crystal establishes a channel to work harmoniously with the people you encounter on a day to day basis.

●**Amber**: This crystal has been used by humans since 8,000 BCE. This crystal is transparent, carrying the light of the sun. It is a very lightweight crystal producing abundance and warmth, promoting many health benefits such as improving mental, emotional, and physical health. It is a great crystal to carry if you are feeling ashamed for something you have done because this crystal allows the being to be comfortable with the acceptance so that you can see the bright side of the future. Real amber is at least 100,000 years old. They come in golden to yellow-orange shades. They are widely available, but the finest comes from Poland. The crystals provide confidence and can help in releasing stress.

●**Banded Agate**: It is also known as Shiva's eyes. These crystals remove inner conflict while harmonizing the body. It also helps in detoxification, enhancing the cellular memory and oxygenation in the cell. If these crystals are placed around a room, they can provide a protective shield in that environment by alleviating negative energies.

•**Topaz**: This word may have come from a Sanskrit word meaning 'fire.' Historical sources have found that the topaz stones refract the colour if placed near poison, so it was kept by kings and queens who feared any kind of deceit and treason. This crystal tunes the vibrancy of your soul and brings abundance and joy in your life. This crystal helps you to live according to your visions, rather than following other people. It also helps you to live with the truth. The colour of this crystal ranges from gold to peachy orange.

•**Garnet**: This crystal is used to neutralize poison, calm fever, and reduce depression. These red stones are regarded as having anti-inflammatory properties, while the yellow stones of this kind provide a remedy against jaundice. Water-infused garnet eases with digestion. Today, the workers who use crystals to heal someone uses garnet crystals to heal heart problems, also, rejuvenate the body. These crystals are also known for amplifying the energy vibration of other crystals so that it can do a regeneration grid: fastening the creating of new cells. In early days, people used to wear the red garnet crystals called that time as carbuncles. With the help of these crystals, people used to convert resentment, pain, or any disease into well-being. Garnet makes you self-aware about your inner world, reflecting where you are self-sabotaging yourself, or resisting change. This crystal gives the right kind of courage to deal with yourself so that you can transform better. This type of crystal is usually suitable for sensitive people; it provides faithfulness to their purpose. These crystals vary from red-orange to vibrant orange.

●**Quartz**: These crystals allow the body to be in balance and tries to calm any disease. Most of the benefits of quartz relate to the proper regulation of the blood pressure, regeneration of cells, and reoxygenation of the tissues in our body. Quartz also affects metabolism. It allows the body to maintain the metabolism well while strengthening the joints, also, producing elasticity. It also takes care of the blood vessels and is anti-inflammatory. Historically, this crystal was also used to be in the cradles of a new-born baby, so that they can connect with the earth. Large quartz was found in the temple of Egyptians which was 8,000 years old. This fascinating quartz also helps to restore the body's vibration. These crystals have black star-like colours in them, a tiny dot, accompanied by white shades of crystals.

●**Rhodonite**: As these types of crystals contain manganese, it encourages the growth of bone structure in the human body. The name of this crystal comes from a Greek word called rosy. They are often of intense bi-colours of black and white. They can restore the emotional balance inside of the human being, also, alleviating the self-destructive tendencies that one has. It promotes brotherhood and lets you see all sides so that if any problems occur, this crystal allows you to see both sides. This crystal allows oneself to feel that all the negative energy is a time-waster. It is also used to heal the bite caused by an insect; this crystal is an effective wound healer. It is said that if someone lies on the rhodonite grid, that person easily get rids of the memory of emotional abuse, replace it with forgiveness and love. If an individual lacks trust in himself/herself, rhodonite provides the needed confidence and unconditional love and acceptance as it supports you through tough situations, helping you to stay calm and heart-centred. They come in white and pink bands, sometimes enveloped in white colours, and sometimes, opaque to magenta.

•**Celestite**: It is an important crystal for cosmic connection. Coming in an ethereal blue form, this crystal offers hope while instilling a wide sense of peace in yourself, expanding your consciousness to promoting the flow of your harmonious existence throughout the whole universe.

This crystal may have minute traces of gold. It sparks the spirit with a good amount of fire, creating that power in the heart. This crystal get rids of the diseases that may be related to genes, embedding the cells with positive vibration to create an order. These crystals also help to relax the muscle tension, while healing any kind of throat conditions.

•**Diamond**: This is the hardest crystal that has even walked the earth. Known for its invincibility gesture, this crystal provides the individual unconquerable force. Diamond's elements are not made on earth. They have come from outer space, revealing those cosmic roots. They are the symbol of eternity and purity. Diamonds have the notion that they have the power to get rid of the wild distractions that humans have, and also, get rids of the senseless fear that the mind sometimes have. Diamond-infused water was the medicine in ancient times that treated jaundice, apoplexy, gallstones, and fevers. On the mental level, diamond crystals provide clarity and allow the mind to stimulate its imagination properly. Diamonds also protect against the electromagnetic frequencies, while helping the individual during stress. It is said that diamonds give the needed patience in expanding consciousness.

●**Turquoise**: The Egyptian goddess Hathor—this crystal was sacred to her. This crystal provides calmness to the soul. It is the bringer of luck and peace. This crystal is considered a fortunate crystal for singers and actors. It is also considered as a powerful counterpart to the evil eye. A turquoise that has been given by a loving and good vibration carry hand creates good fortune and happiness. This saying has been taken from an Arabic proverb. It is used to heal sore throats and headaches. This crystal is said to lose its colour whenever the crystal is in the presence of illness or evils. It also carries anti-inflammatory elements within it, helping in cramps and arthritis. If you want to release your mental exhaustion and physical pain, wear this crystal. It is said that this crystal also helps in depression. It contains phosphoric acid, this is how the water-induced base clears the sore throat. These crystals also contain traces of iron, have protective qualities, and may also have copper in it. Turquoise also helps the pessimistic individual, allowing that person to feel that he/she should seek answers rather than focussing on the problems. It alleviates the negative belief patterns and gets rid of the toxins caused by those negative beliefs, enhancing the human learning experience. These stones come in bright blue to glowing light green.

•**Sapphire**: This crystal is of high potency in Vedic astrology. It symbolizes the importance of light, that the light is there in the darkness. It preserves joy, courage, and the heart while pleasing the important senses. In the times of Ezekiel, sapphires crystals were used to form the throne of God. It is used to heal the diseases relating to blood while regulating the overacting glands. Also, sapphires are good for improving the elasticity of the veins. They are also very sovereign for the sight. They usually come in a deep blue colour.

- **Hanksite**: This stone comes from the muddy depths of the Californian lake. This crystal symbolizes the need for the soul to scratch its depth through the karmic past. In Hanksite crystals, Halite is a component that is embedded in it—a type of purifier that cleans the energy that disturbs the spiritual calmness. It clears all the negative energy while enhancing your aura. If someone had a power struggle in the past, this crystal helps the individual to accept that through forgiveness. Hanksite grids are required in the toxic places to clean the environment so that an individual can be free from his inside pollution and the pollution around him or her. This crystal helps to get rid of fluid retention. While it helps in enhancing the cellular memory too, Hanksite crystals also assist in cleansing the lymphatic system through positive vibrations. If you have breathing difficulties, hold this crystal on your chest. The inflammation is caused by the mucus membrane, holding Hanksire will help the chest to heal. This crystal blocks bad emotions and turns into forgiveness.

These crystals colour ranges from pale yellow to greyish-green.

●**Beryl**: It symbolizes everlasting youth and happiness. This crystal helps in healing eye problems. Historically, this crystal was rubbed on an individual's swollen throat to cure quinsy. This crystal was also placed over the liver to get rid of the pain associated with the liver. The modern-day crystal workers use beryl-induced water to heal their sore throat via gargles. This crystal also helps in detoxification, allowing the crystal to cope up with the stress by placing the crystal over to the liver or lymphatic system. This crystal strengthens the circulation of the blood, and also, strengthens the heart and lung. This crystal is excellent for beginners as it helps the learner to clarify the thoughts and alleviates the deeply embedded thoughts that no longer serve you while raising your vibration to follow your soul's path. The pure quality of beryl is colourless but is usually tinted by fake colours.

●**Flint**: This crystal held the fire's essence inside it without which life wasn't possible.

Historically, this crystal was used to open the portals between different words and provided the tools to negotiate with other worlds. This was written in a resonant stone. This crystal enhances the path of spiritual enlightenment. It also balances the masculinity and femininity powers to convert into a sacred inner marriage. This crystal cleanses the different chakras (later in this book) and helps in creating a different aura in an individual. This crystal also helps in treating the ulcers and the troubles with the joint. The power of this crystal creates a vibration that assists in healing the individual's spiritual, emotional, and psychological realms. Flint crystals also helps to find the underlying causes of depression by bringing your thoughts into conscious awareness. Their colours vary in dark grey, black, or brown.

●**Zincite**: These crystals come in a different range of colours with different frequencies. A natural zincite is rare and is formed inside fiery chimneys of smelting plants. This crystal is for those who want to get in tune with their gut instincts through the signals of their body; a great deal of intuition comes naturally through it. Wearing Zincite crystals will alert you to those instincts. This crystal helps you to get rid of those unconscious mental influences that control an individual's behaviour. They are those hypnotic commands that are set by other people whom you don't agree with. Zincite crystals help the person to get close with like-minded people. These crystals help in shock and trauma. These crystals contain zinc which is good for teeth, cellular metabolism, hair, bones, and skin. It also takes care of the joints. To examine different effects of this stone, an individual must have different zincite crystal colours. Red zincite energises and provides stability to the structure. Green and yellow zincite crystals provide calm and the initiation of the process where different rebalances are required. It also gets rid of the negative patterns in the body that make the way for the diseases.

How to choose the right crystals?

Choosing the right kind of crystal is very important for an individual. It is like developing a personal relationship with the stones. You maybe are drawn toward crystal, or maybe you want to purchase crystals for a friend, or a family, or just are curious to have them at your home. There are several ways to choose the right kinds of crystals. Firstly, use your intuition. Secondly, use your logic. And third, use the combination of these two things. Or you may be into arts and you want a nice collection of crystals. It all depends on your viewpoint: what do you think about them? What made them grasp you? Why are you curious about them? You have to listen to your inner self. You may find yourself greatly attracted to a particular type of crystal. Or you just decided to choose the stones by their properties. The same thing can be said about its shapes and sizes. There are times in your life where you find yourself lost; you are emotionally damaged, psychologically frustrated, and want a better life. As the properties of the crystals are already discussed in this book, from reading it you can make your choices. You can shortlist your crystals. You have to trust the universe if you are not sure about your choices. You have to close your eyes, have to take a deep breath and have to ask the universe to help you. Once you are through with it, gather your stones. Spread them a few inches away and place your arm at each crystal. Feel the vibration. See for yourself what works for you and what doesn't. You may find that there may be more than one crystal you like. Take those crystals. They are right for you.

There may be some instances where you may have a dream about crystals. Don't neglect that dream. It is the message sent by your subconscious mind to work with that energy. You need to decipher your dream: reflect on it as soon as you wake up. Start writing journals on it and how you react to the dream emotionally. Try to remember the symbols in your dream with the crystal that you have dreamed about. Check if some objects stand out—book, elephant, number-letter, or symbols like OM sign, it can be anything. Or there may be archetypes in your dream state—deities, ascended masters, angels, or any strong inspiration in the modern age. Each association of the objects in your dream, including the crystal, you can compare these two things, and try to find some cues because each archetype has some symbolic meaning attached to it, some energy qualities that you can see in the stone. Or there can be instances where you may receive crystals or crystal as a gift. If someone receives a crystal, the receiver is chosen and can amplify the energy of the crystal. You can later reflect on why you were chosen for this gift. You can reflect on the intuition of the person who has presented this gift to you. To prepare for the stone, your insights are valuable. And if you are choosing for someone else, your insights are still valuable too. First, you need to visualize the person with different crystals. You need to react to the crystals in regards to that person and see where your heart goes. Another method would require you to close your eyes and see how the crystals respond to the person who you are going to present your gift to.

To get the right crystals, you need to select the right store for your stones. To get them, you need to think about their chemical structures, their vibrational frequencies, and their energy fields, so in the end, choosing a right crystal, there is nothing right and wrong in it. But be aware of the fake crystals. These days, fake crystals are flooding the market. People love crystals because they contain energy. For this perfectness, things cannot be replicated. To spot fake crystals, the first thing you can do is to educate yourself. So, read this book. Read and learn that natural crystals can change their appearance, fake crystals cannot. Real crystals can also develop fractures, their colours can change. They can also fade. Natural crystals are found in nature, while the synthetic crystals have the same chemical, visual, and physical properties. Some crystals are aligned with your goals and some crystals are aligned with your chakras (discussed later in the book). To buy the right crystal for you, you can also make a choice based on their forms. There are three types of common crystals—raw, cut and tumbled. Raw comes straight away from the earth. They are less expensive and many people want the natural appearance of these crystals. While the cut crystals come in many shapes such as cubes, wands, points, etc. The shape has nothing to do with the physical properties of the crystals. Whereas, tumble crystals are tiny in size and are polished alternatively. They are great if you want to carry these crystals in your pocket. They are also less expensive compared to cut crystals and are a perfect way for the beginners to start their journey with crystals.

How to use crystals?

There are many ways to use the different types of crystals, but it all comes down to your personal preference. Some crystals are worn close to the body and some are used as jewelleries. Even if you don't have enough knowledge about crystals, you will automatically choose jewellery because they are more regarded as a fashionable thing. As already mentioned, you should select the crystals which are personal to you and what your intuition tells you. Crystals close to your body are usually used for healing or protection. They tend to have their effect all over the body. This happens because the stones close to your body creates a high vibrational field. And also, if put on the specific places, it can help the area to heal faster. The energies of the crystal are usually travelled to where they are needed. You can efficiently direct the energy to your body if the stone is in your pocket, or if you are wearing a necklace, or a ring. The length of the chain, embedded in it the crystals also determine the effect on the different chakras.

The other method of using crystal is when you are bathing. You can either place the crystals inside the water or around the bathtub. When you are bathing, it is a cleansing act. Having crystals around you can help you to get rid of your stress by each wash, also, helping you with the exhaustion that you have experienced during the day while removing your negative emotions. Crystals help in soaking in the negativity so that they can never return. The healing energy of the stone will go where it is needed. The best crystal to use in this method is Rose Quartz.

The next method would involve using the crystals by placing them under the pillow. Crystals help to combat insomnia and provides a night of good quality sleep. Psychic attacks, sleep paralysis, and nightmares—crystals also help to get rid of these things while assuring you that you get a good night sleep. Good sleep leads to balanced hormonal levels, stress-free day, good mood, and good digestion because the immune system is strong. Crystals with the sleep are like a bonus. It also can help you to remember your dream, while taking you to other out of the world kind of experiences, helping you to fight nightmares.

You can even place the crystals around your home, so that you can change the atmosphere of life around you, to get rid of those negative energies. Raw crystals and crystal clusters are better because they are big, covering space better, giving a greater energy field. These crystals can catch negative energy faster and can promote harmony around the environment. On the other hand, the formulation of the crystals also depicts a certain order which helps in quiet down the body, while enhancing its function. If you can change your thought process and try to focus on the solutions that can be solved, then crystals can come in handy, especially, during meditation. You can place the stone on your hands, holding them calmly, while you are meditating.

Crystals can also help in cleaning the environment around you. If the environment is polluted, which it is, you are polluted, but you can take steps to counter the pollution. Microwaves, radio waves, wi-fi, and plastic, these things harm us. They overload our body with different stresses. Ever wondered about why there is so much peace in the agricultural area, and so much noise in the urban areas? Too much stress can cause us to have diseases and illnesses. The natural energy of the earth gets surrounded everywhere, but the artificial built-in nature, it distorts those frequencies. Crystals to counteract the pollution—mental, emotional, or manifesting outside—can help us to increase our energy frequencies to counteract society positively. That's why crystals are gaining popularity amidst the presence of computers, metals, artificial lightings, cars, air conditioners, etc.

How to make crystals more effective?

Crystals are a powerful amplifier of great vibrational energies. When you combine them with certain things such as affirmations, programming, healing mantras, and combining different crystals—these transformative abilities provide opportunities for positive transformation. Affirmations are very important in your life. You share with yourself what you really want, intently. You create a conscious statement in your reality to achieve your dreams with the help of the crystals. Adding affirmations in it is like giving a message to the universe because the universe listens. It operates in an algorithm of cosmic waves reacting with the vibrations of the stones. With the universe, you communicate your goals, visions, wishes, needs, wants, etc. When you want to manifest your reality with affirmations and with the help of crystals, the vibrational field of your life automatically gets changed and gets put on a higher level. But first, let's understand the difference between programming your crystals, and when using affirmations. Many people use programming with their crystals to suit their specific purposes. This makes sense, but this method might become restrictive. The limitation comes when you set your crystal for just a specific purpose. That direct objective might hinder the full potentiality of the crystal. But with affirmation, you are not setting any limitations or direct objective. You are allowing the crystals to work with your being, your soul. Stones know the way to heal the individuals who own them, and here, you are not imposing anything but just working with the crystal with the free flow of your energy because you will not all the time will be aware of what's happening to your body, the direction of your mind, body, and soul. That's the reality of life. You are incorporation crystals to help you move ahead in your life with courage and determination. Crystals are a way to find out the deep layers within yourself, but at the end of the day, you are the one who has to do the work.

There are also other ways to make stones more effective in its healing power. Crystal mantras are an effective way to increase the level of your healing. So, let's just dive into it. "I encourage positive change and share my talents with the world" –self-explanatory, eh? But which stone to choose? Citrine is one of the crystals that lets you live in the moment. It raises your self-esteem and confidence and gives you the power to manifest your reality with your full potential. This crystal is associate with a prosperity consciousness. It provides you that mental and emotional focus to increase your skills; hence, the various talents. More than the power of intention, Citrine lets you recognize your inner riches and allows you to trust the universe to provide you with that enigma to achieve anything in life. It opens your mind to attract new possibilities.

The next mantra is, "I open myself up to the transformation and invoke the manifestation of my highest destiny." You know a giant meteor has hit the earth eleven million years ago into a glass-like substance. This crystal was Moldavite. These crystals are very good for expanding consciousness and are a great source for transforming oneself. Containing within itself a very high vibrational frequency, many people feel a surge of rush in their bodies when they have Moldavite with them. They are the great crystals that allow you to focus your attention on the cause, trying to solve the imbalances inside you. Some other crystals may be needed with Moldavite because using this crystal alone would cause dizziness. This stone can provide the cosmic energy down to your physical body so that you can feel aligned with the vibrational frequency of the earth to feel at home.

"I'm happy. I'm surrounded by friends and family that support my happiness." Blue Lace Agate is a great source for peace of mind. These crystals are said to open the throat chakra, so that free flow of thoughts, expressions, and feelings that had once been blocked spread easily. Psychosomatic throat problems create a blockage of the right flow of communication, Blue Lace Agate is a great crystal to alleviate that blockage. With the help of it, providing you with that ability to speak, this crystal brings the supportive people around you such as family and friends, so that you can maintain a proper balance around all aspects of life. Blue Lace Agate restores that vibrational energy to the thyroid and parathyroid glands, also, helping the metabolism in your body to function properly.

"I'm unique. I'm amazing." This is the easiest mantra you can remember if you have an Amethyst crystal. This meaning of this word is 'freedom from harm' and 'sincerity'. Historically, this stone was worn by royalties. It symbolizes deep love, wisdom, peace of mind, and devotion. The legend says that this crystal protected against drunkenness. This crystal is also worn in Christian churches to signify victory over passion and spiritual power. The vibration of this crystal removes subtle diseases. In ancient times, Amethyst was used to heal headaches, but in today's world, this stone is used to calm anxiety, while getting rid of psychological and physical pain. Amethyst helps in creating that needed balance in hormone production. This crystal might help in psychosomatic problems by easing the digestive system. This stone helps in absorbing the negativity around you to provide your body that needed stress-free balance.

The next method to make crystals more effective would be using various crystals together: to combine them to amplify the capabilities of stones so that a powerful transformation can take place. For example, take Chrysocolla. This crystal is a very powerful detoxifier and can get rid of many cramps to ensure you a good night sleep. It helps you to move away with egocentricity. This stone also assists you in stimulating the throat, eyes, and your overall metabolism. If you combine this crystal with Smokey quartz, this combination can help you to clear the fungal infection. A strong energizer for the psyche and the body, it resolves the recklessness installed in every human being, transforming it at a greater level. It also helps in stimulating the liver function. The other crystal would be Hanksite, which we have already talked about. If you combine this crystal with Lemurian seed crystals, it helps to stabilize the healing grids. If you can place these stones at your feet, it helps in clearing out all the negativity. You just have to cleanse the stone as often as you can during the use. As Hanksite also contains Halite, this crystal easily disintegrates. With the remnants, you can either bury it under the water to detoxify the environment, or you can bury under the ground. Morganite is another crystal known for providing emotional stability. If you combine this crystal with Azeztulite, your repressed internal conflict gets healed. Tanzanite is another crystal that you can combine it with Danburite and Iolite so that you can initiate the process of karmic healing. Tanzanite helps people to get out of their stress zones. Iolite crystals are the source for opening the portal of intuition, helping in clearing the vision. It also helps in determining the cause of addiction that you might have. While clearing the thoughts, it helps you to express your true self. Whereas, Danburite opens the heart chakra. It helps the individual to learn the art of acceptance. For its metaphysical properties, it helps in relieving the emotional pain. Combining these crystals: Tanzanite, Iolite, and Danburite—they provide the gateway to real karmic healing.

Chapter 2: Here Are 8 Useful Remedies To Cure Yeast Infection

When you don't have a clue, yeast contaminations are brought about by the microorganisms Candida Albicans. The microbes dwell in our bodies and are generally innocuous. In any case, when there is a noteworthy unevenness in our body, the microorganisms develop and results in contamination. So you have to fix the candida contamination usually.

Here are eight helpful solutions to fix Yeast contamination.

1. Hydrate - our body needs a ton of water to work appropriately, and one of those capacities is to expel poisons. If the body isn't hydrated adequately, the microorganisms can develop much quicker.

2. Use Tea Tree Oil - Tea tree oil is known for is hostile to bacterial properties; you can straightforwardly apply this to the contaminated zone to bring alleviation.

3. Aloe Vera - as far back as Egyptian occasions, the aloe vera plant has been utilized for it against contagious properties. You can go it to glue and legitimately apply to the contaminated territory.

4. Eat Garlic - garlic isn't just for battling vampires, the counter bacterial properties of garlic are likewise useful for evacuating the disease.

5. Utilize hostile to contagious herbs in your eating regimen - you can include herbs with the high enemy of bacterial properties to your supper like oregano, garlic, and olive oil.

6. Expel sugar - expel sugar from your diet, as this indeed triggers the development of the microscopic organisms. Attempt to likewise decrease your admission of bread and sustenances wealthy in sugars.

7. Wear-free dress - at times, microscopic organisms develop in our body on account of the garments we wear. Attempt to wear garments that are agreeable and not to tight in the body.

8. Exercise - by practicing we evacuate all the undesirable poisons in our body by perspiring, this additionally incorporates the microscopic organisms that cause the disease.

Useful Remedies to Get Rid of Acne

Nobody likes acne, and when you've it you might want to find the best cure as fast as feasible. Other individuals are in all likelihood not as concentrated on your acne as you're, even though it might perhaps make you reluctant. You shouldn't endure it, either, so here are some effective acne solutions for the endeavor.

You can discover bunches of reasons for grown-up acne. However, some of them are less hard to manage than other individuals. When you are a lady, it's reachable that any acne you've maybe an inadequate response to the makeup you wear, which could be incredible news just because all you'll do to clear up your issue is switch beautifiers. A portion of the lower quality beautifying agents, for instance, will contain harsh synthetics that have been perceived to trigger a few folks to experience the ill effects of acne. When you accept this could be causing your acne, supplant your present make-up with unadulterated caused make-to up. Hormones may likewise bring about grown-up acne in females, and this is typically brought about by anti-conception medication pills. So for adult women, a direct acne treatment could be to roll out some simple improvements.

A new unadulterated solution for acne is taking an olive leaf. It truly is ideal for making this strong enemy of the parasitic plant in enhancement structure. Olive leaf can effectively execute the microorganisms or infections that will bring about acne. Taking it with your other acne cures can support their adequacy. The wellbeing preferences for your total body make using olive leaf every day an extraordinary idea.

Sound fat is only one strategy to manage acne. Solid fat like fish oil is an excellent method for diminishing the irritation that causes your acne. Different dinners which are high in sound Omega fat comprise of nuts like almonds, pecans and cashews, avocados and olive oil. You have likewise to remove care to remain from dinners containing unhealthy trans fat, which means scanning for suppers which may be thoroughly free of hydrogenated oils. The sorts of fat that you eat can help or damage your skin and eating just the solid fat might be a fantastic way to deal with usually fix your acne.

Disposing of acne is hugely a rigorous methodology; however, not an unthinkable one. Various folks surrender too rapidly or don't allow a particular treatment adequate time to work. These cures have been gainful for different people, yet you'll endeavor them to find if they can work for you.

Useful Remedies For Athlete's Foot Infection

Competitor's foot is usually caused as a result of dermatophytes (contagious contamination), which likewise has the therapeutic name tinea pedis. The parasite causing competitor's foot often happens when strolling with uncovered feet in warm and moist spots, similar to regular showers and storage spaces, which are perfect spots for contagious reproducing.

The parasite twists and breeds effectively if the foot isn't kept in a sterile way. The dead cells in the skin are left in the foot by the parasite, and the foot contamination is seen later.

As the contamination spreads, the encompassing foot skin turns out to be textured and dry. As the contamination spread rankles, irritation effectively creates. The rankles that are in the midst of the toes break and open the skin to give severe agony and a consuming sensation. The puss discharged by the messed up rankles additionally makes the contamination spread quicker. Another side effect of a competitor's foot is irritation on the skin bordering the rile, which is problematic and exasperating.

Competitor's foot is reparable as different powerful medications are accessible. Medication stores supply hostile to parasitic meds, which fix a competitor's foot totally and successfully. Some oral applications and topical creams are additionally available to apply on foot to strip from foot disease. Aside from these specific home cures are likewise accessible to fix competitor's foot.

Various home cures are accessible to stay away from the tedious and disturbing contagious ailments like competitor's foot. The best relieving drug is available in your kitchen compartments and its garlic. Squashed garlic can be kept on dry socks, which are worn while dozing. This gives extraordinary help and remedy for the infection. Numerous fundamental oils help to fix a competitor's foot. Tea tree oil is the most regular and standard treatment for this parasitic ailment. It has a huge enemy of contagious property, which is best contrasted with different drugs. Applying the oil on the tainted region of your skin regularly for seven days will take out the foot contamination.

Some Useful Remedies For Candida

There are many solutions for candida which can be compelling and help you to beat common side effects, for example, tingling and general distress. Many individuals will encounter this sooner or later in their lives; however, fortunately, it is something which we know a ton about and can be treated in various extraordinary and viable ways.

The reason it happens is because of an irregularity in microorganisms, which makes yeast develop and spread. The best alternative that you have accessible to you is to neutralize this by using various systems available to you. These are regularly minor changes you can make to your way of life, which will have a significant effect.

Sugar advances the development of yeast in the body just as prompting a scope of wellbeing concerns which can detrimentally affect the body. This is commonly found in nibble nourishments, for example, sweet and cakes and this way it is astute to diminish your utilization of these. This will likewise beneficially affect your weight too.

This is additionally obvious with regards to liquor. Notwithstanding being made fundamentally from handled sugars, it regularly contains yeast alongside next to no in the method for dietary benefits and many void calories. When you drink liquor all the time, at that point, attempt to diminish your utilization to have any effect with issues of this sort, and this will demonstrate supportive alongside different solutions for a candida.

Having enough water in your framework consistently causes your body to be sound and adjusted, and this encourages you to check any diseases and for the most part, be a more advantageous individual. Take a stab at drinking at least eight glasses per day and don't substitute it with different refreshments as these don't have the equivalent helpful effect that plain water has. Your body will thank you, and it will likewise notably affect your skin tone and assimilation.

A reliable and adjusted eating routine will give you a superior shot of managing issues of this sort. Furthermore, it will assist you with having a more advantageous immune framework and also give your body the supplements and nutrients that it needs if it will stay free of contamination and ready to manage any future diseases.

Wearing tight-fitting garments makes it increasingly plausible that issues of this benevolent will influence you. Change what you wear and furthermore take a gander at utilizing unscented cleansers and cleansing agents as these are known to exasperate conditions like candida. This additionally applies to any cleanliness items which are vigorously perfumed that you happen to utilize.

When things are as yet not improving having attempted these solutions for candida, at that point, you should take a brief trip and see a specialist who will analyze you and blueprint every single potential choice you have accessible for treatment. Conversing with them can give you a scope of thoughts that will assist you with preventing this occurrence again, and they may recommend you with something that will handle the issue.

Helpful Remedies For Constipation

Solutions for stoppage are helpful when there is a need to calm one's self from troublesome and difficult stool discharges. Unpredictable bowel movement isn't a confusion or infection; however, it is a common condition related to the section of dry and hard dung and deficient departure of the bowel. This issue should be tended to as ahead of schedule as conceivable to keep away from the beginning of ailments brought upon by the maintenance of nourishment in the bowel.

What are the prescribed obstruction cures?

There are a few over-the-counter treatments accessible anyway there are symptoms related with them. A specific strategy for getting help from this issue is best liked. The following are a couple of conventional techniques you should need to attempt. Some might be well-known, and others may not.

Leafy foods are fiber-rich, so they can help in framing cumbersome and delicate stools that are anything but difficult to pass. For roughage, eat pears, mangoes, oranges, sweet potatoes, carrots, and peas.

Garlic may not be your first decision but rather its high potassium substance helps in appropriate intestinal muscle constrictions that increments peristaltic movement. Without a doubt help, add garlic to soup, nectar or squeeze and have it three times each day. It is safe to say that you are experiencing ceaseless bowel movement issues?

Aloe Vera juice invigorates bowel movements and is best when encountering constant bowel discharge challenges. Likewise, prune juice is a characteristic purgative that mellows the stool for a better bowel movement.

Increment your admission of Vitamin C to help your free framework. A decent source is a lemon juice blended with warm water. Taste this without salt or sugar.

Besides these solutions for obstruction, ensure that you likewise have a reasonable eating routine and drink a lot of water. Exercise is additionally great assistance in managing bowel movements.

Useful Remedies For Kidney Stones - Waiting For Your Kidney Stones to Pass is a Thing of the Past

There are a lot of useful solutions for kidney stones! In any case, most specialists suggest drinking a lot of water and pausing and pausing and pausing. There is a motivation behind why they guide you to pause.

Certainty! In about 85% of kidney stone cases, the stones usually are little enough to go during pee. This will, in all probability, occur within four days of the side effects. Also, side effects for kidney stones incorporate a severe agony in the crotch, back or side. The best treatment for these side effects is to drink a lot of water to enable the kidney to stone pass. Most specialists prescribe drinking 2 to 3 quarts for every day and suggest taking agony executioners. Is there more you can do?

Definitely! Furthermore, you may end up disillusioned with your primary care physician's recommendation once you hear some other useful solutions for kidney stones.

Powerful Natural Remedies for Kidney Stones

Kidney stones hurt. Many ladies who have had children state that kidney stone torment can be more regrettable than pregnancy. However, you don't need to manage the agony for longer than 24 hours. Did you realize that 90% of kidney stones should go within the first 24 hours of treatment when you utilize a couple of standard solutions for break down them? Here are some useful and successful tips for beginning your treatment today.

1. Aversion and treatment more often than not walk connected at the hip. With collective wellbeing, you can, for the most part, fix most infirmities by treating the reason. In this way, you ought to drink water (ideally refined) because lack of hydration is ordinarily the reason for most calcium-based kidney stones.

2. You should, likewise remain dynamic. It is demonstrated that a robust and influential body works all the more

effectively. All your real indications, including your kidneys, will work better. Along these lines, take that walk you appear to never possess energy for. Get up early tomorrow to go to the wellness focus. It could help flush your stones.

3. You ought to likewise maintain a strategic distance from every single zesty sustenance until your stones pass. An ongoing report demonstrated how kidney stones are practically nonexistent to those societies who eat no fiery foods.

4. You ought to likewise drink foods grown from the ground squeezes, for example, carrot, grape, and orange juices. These juices contain high degrees of citrates. Citrates decrease the development of uric corrosive and help wipe out the arrangement of calcium salts (most kidney stones are comprised of calcium).

5. You ought to likewise take a magnesium supplement of no under 300-350 mg for every day. Many kidney stones sufferers are inadequate in magnesium, and enhancement could also help in passing your stones.

6. At long last, phosphoric corrosive has additionally demonstrated to be useful in dissolving kidney stones. Phosphoric corrosive is consumable and is found in everything from sodas to cleaning items. This caustic gives drinks a citrusy taste and is likewise sufficiently able to expel calcium from baths and showers.

Step by step instructions to Get Rid of Blackheads - 3 Useful Remedies on How to Get Rid of Blackheads!

Many individuals utilize a clogged pore extractor as a guide for this issue; indeed, they can work for a few; however, chances are the zits you evacuated will return, perhaps more. So give these cures a shot and perceive how they work...

Nectar

Warm some nectar and spot it on the zits for 10-15 minutes at that point, wash it off. I have perused many audits many individuals guaranteeing this cure is the ideal approach to expel zits so I gave it a shot myself and I should state it was viable.

Rose and Oatmeal Mask

This treatment is incredible to dispose of the clogged pores you as of now have and avert future breakouts. Blend oats powder with rose water to make a glue and Spread the paste all over with fingertips and enable it to sit for 10-15 minutes before washing off with virus water.

Heating Soda and Water

Blend 3-4 tablespoons of heating soft drink with 3-4 tablespoons of water. Rub this arrangement on your skin for a couple of minutes, and flush with warm water. This cure on the best way to dispose of clogged pores might be potent, and it comes highly suggested by many.

Dermatitis In Children - Useful Remedies To Beat Eczema

There are three sorts of rashes that children will, in general, create. When the reason isn't chicken pox or toxic substance ivy, it must be skin inflammation. In such a case, the skin will turn textured, red, and it will create bruises. If the tingling surpasses a breaking point, the skin will begin shedding as scales. Dermatitis is otherwise called Dermatitis. Dermatitis means skin irritation, and here the skin will in general, turn sore and pink. This is an extremely regular issue. It has been discovered that one in every ten youngsters will in broad experience the ill effects of this issue, and this is beneath the age gathering of five. When the kid turns into an adolescent, there are fewer odds of this issue happening.

Dry skin is only one of the issues that dermatitis makes, and the other is the way that the surface will, in general, tingle horribly. Skin inflammation is constant, and it can happen intermittently. An extraordinary sort of cell that is available in the body will respond to any foreign entity that interacts with the skin. Here the skin aggravation happens to secure it. A portion of the external agencies that are unsafe may make the skin over-respond as they trigger out the response in self-protection. This can make the skin sore, red, and irritated. These abnormal cells are available in considerable amounts in youngsters who have skin inflammation.

For the most part, if illnesses like asthma, general sensitivities, or feed fever are available in the family, the child has a higher possibility of getting skin inflammation. This issue is passed down from the guardians and is available in the qualities. Scientists have discovered that children who have skin inflammation have littler odds of creating roughage fever or asthma further down the road. One beneficial thing about skin inflammation is that it isn't infectious. Numerous indications help in recognizing skin inflammation. The most important is the rash. At first, it may appear as though the outbreaks are vanishing, yet they are sure to return. Even though skin inflammation rashes are known to tingle gravely, this need not be the situation consistently. These rashes invariably begin from inside the elbows and behind the knees and after that progressively spread to the next body parts.

There are numerous different sorts of rashes that can be shaped other than skin inflammation; just a specialist would commonly have the option to recognize a typical rash from dermatitis. When it is affirmed that the outbreaks are because of dermatitis, the youngster should utilize salves or saturating creams to prevent the skin from drying and furthermore to stop the irritation. When the explosions don't stop the specialist may recommend corticosteroids. This can be as cream or treatment, which must be connected to control the anger of the skin. Antihistamine can likewise be taken for severe swelling. This is accessible in either as a fluid or as a pill. The specialists will endorse an anti-microbial when the tingling has created contamination.

Certain substances trigger skin inflammation. Youngsters who are inclined to skin inflammation ought to dodge these substances. These substances could be cleansers, cleansers, hot and sweat-soaked skin, dry air (during winters), and scents. Skin bothering can increment when it interacts with certain textures or residue parasites. Regardless of whether there is extreme tingling, the youngster must avoid scratching it seriously since it will just purpose the skin to tingle more and it will likewise help in spreading disease. If there should be an occurrence of serious scratching the surface can now and again break and drain, and this is the thing that makes the contamination spread. The best solution for this is to wet fabric with cold water and spot it on the zone where there is severe tingling. Guardians ought to guarantee that the nails of the kids are sliced short to stay away from the skin from tearing when the tyke scratches it. In particular, the patient should drink loads of water since this aids in keeping the skin soggy.

Have You Ever Wondered About The Power Of Healing Crystals?

The reason for utilizing recuperating precious stones is to reestablish the equalization of inconspicuous energies and to restore the physical creature being to a solid-state. Precious stones and Gemstones are one of the most lovely, enchanted and significant "vitality medication" devices, which have been utilized for a considerable length of time all through all societies, religions, and realms. With the more grounded requirement for non-physical mending joined with physical recuperating, numerous individuals are finding the intensity of extraordinary recuperating precious stones. Gems are utilized in reflection and profound services, laid on the body during sorts of back rub or bodywork when an individual is resting, or put in drinking or washing waters. Gems bring incredible advantages to the recuperating field.

Precious stones, gemstones, and minerals can be useful assets in showing us how to recuperate ourselves. Precious stones are found in all shapes, sizes, hues, and synthesis. Their related recuperating properties can choose precious stones, or they can be selected by the shading that is related with the Chakra overseeing the particular affliction, malady, issue or aspect of your life that necessities adjusting or mending. Precious stones of different hues help in the recuperating procedure by making certain tranquil feelings and changing the perspective.

The emotions and instincts you get might be unobtrusive, it won't resemble a "blast of firecrackers," however when you begin confiding in yourself and your sentiments, your internal direction will get more grounded, and you will intuitively know/feel what to do or which recuperating gems to use at which times. You will find out about recuperating precious stones by focusing on how they affect you. The voyage you start to go with recovering precious stones will change your life perpetually, and you will develop to cherish them as they upgrade your reality and help you on all levels.

A couple of the various sorts of recuperating precious stones to attempt may include:

Agates - help the wearer feel ensured and are particularly compelling for kids. They likewise help to focus your considerations and feelings.

Amethyst - viable for uneasiness or melancholy and cerebral pains/headaches, bring quietness and quiet during contemplation, is viewed as a Master Healing Stone.

Chakras - advantage brain, body and soul and prompts a more prominent feeling of harmony and internal parity

Rose Quartz - extraordinary for enthusiastic recuperating, love, magnificence, quietness, excusing, consideration and confidence

Use them in the manner that feels directly for you - hold them, lay down with them, place them in your home, wear them....after this is your adventure and all life is valuable, and this incorporates the stone spirits of precious stones and minerals, some being recuperating gems and mending minerals. Anyone can rehearse precious stone mending, and to they are appealing around the home, as blessings, or in surprising spots, for example, gardens and fish tanks.

Precious stones have been a significant piece of the recuperating scene insofar as man has strolled upon this world. We would all be able to profit by the intensity of precious stones.

Healing Crystals Being Used by Many for Wellbeing

There have been many types of convictions and faiths among individuals of today, and gem recuperating is a structure which has turned into an exceptionally looked for after idea. The premise of the utilization of precious stones for mending purposes probably won't be comprehended by many. In any case, if this thought is profoundly considered and individuals will attempt to see the support of these, at that point, they will likewise begin putting stock in these items so that there will be many individuals who are having confidence in this arrangement of mending.

Even though there have been built up ways by which individuals put stock in their field of allopathy, homeopathy, and naturopathy, the mending precious stones have come up as a charming astonishment for many. These days, many individuals have begun having confidence in the arrangement of precious stone mending since it tends to be seen that they are enhancing these gems which are being worn with the conviction that these will help avoid a lot of infections.

There is an assortment of precious stones which have mending properties, and these will prompt their buys from various sources. The offers of such mending precious stones have gone up very high as of late, and a lot of it depends on the conviction among individuals, who expect that their illnesses will be recuperated if they wear these gems. Likewise, another viewpoint which can be believed to be prevalent is the ascent of different faith healers, who recommend individuals to wear these sorts of precious stones on their body.

The fierceness of having faith in gem mending has been there since ages. However, they never went to the cutting edge in such an enormous scale as they have in the 21st century. Individuals are taking the responsibility to the assortment of strategies for precious stone recuperating in a meaningful manner. This has to do with the faith in such precious stones among the normal man, who are scanning for such sorts of gems. The evidence of this fame is portrayed in the manner, the closeout of such flowers has expanded in volume and individuals are additionally prepared to pay a decent cost to claim them and use them in their ways of life.

They are scanning for such recuperating gems in the shops, and online stores, and many organizations are likewise publicizing them for the information of the basic man. Such precious stones can be of various shapes and sizes and plans, and every one of them accompanies a lot of confirmations from individuals who guarantee to have researched them. It is accordingly observed that the faith and conviction of individuals have expanded immensely, with the goal that they are purchasing these from whichever source they can discover and after that utilizing it as coordinated. Such a pattern has a lot to do with the faith that individuals have created throughout the years, a component, which must be accepted if they mark the number of individuals wearing such recuperating precious stones.

Chapter 3: Crystals And Crystal Healing

What are Crystals?

A crystal, in the simplest sense, is a piece of homogenous solid material, which naturally consists of a geometrically even structure. Furthermore, its plane faces are proportionally arranged.

Crystals are formed through a natural process called crystallization or solidification. Even so, not all crystals are naturally solid.

Crystals are pure elements. More than that, they are living beings. They are made up of protons, neutrons and electrons that all work to together to create and maintain their geometry.

A crystal's atoms, molecules and ions are sculpted by Mother Nature's fair hand to form a regular and repeating configuration, which spreads to three spatial dimensions. You'll note that this arrangement is visually evident in large crystals like the Quartz. You may also observe this unique structure upon examining smaller stones like the Agate under a microscope.

A crystal's sacred shape is the result of the flawless stacking of its unit cells. Fashioning such a shape will be impossible if there are any gaps.

Are Crystals and Gemstones the Same?

No, they're not. A gemstone is merely a lovely mineral-based stone derived from the earth, which has very little flaws, if any. Gemstones are cut, polished then used as jewelry, décor, or collection. If a gemstone consists of a crystalline structure, it may be categorized as a crystal. An example of which is the diamond. Even so, not all gemstones may be categorized as crystals. Likewise, not all crystals are considered as gemstones. Take amber, for example. Rather than being made up of a mineral base, it is derived from fossilized tree resin, which is an organic base. Mineral-based stones are usually harder than stones made up of other substances.

While gemstones generally have a solid color, crystals are more translucent and lightly colored in comparison. The color of crystals are highly affected by the transmission of light through the rock.

When it comes to pricing, it is necessary to know that precious or semi-precious gemstones, like emeralds, are usually more costly than crystals. The price is typically dependent upon the stone's rarity and other characteristics like cut, hardness, refractive index, specific gravity, luster, color, cleavage and chemical composition. Crystals are less expensive. In fact, not all crystals are considered as precious. Take salt crystals, for instance.

When buying crystals, the main things you need to consider are the atom composition, the shape and the defects. As for investment, most people consider it wise to opt for gemstones with crystalline structures.

What is Crystal Healing?

It is a healing technique that is rapidly regaining its popularity. The truth is that far from being a new age craze, crystal healing can be traced back to ancient civilizations. They were used as beauty aids and were carried as amulets for protection whether from evil spirits or the perils of travel. Simply put, crystal healing is a time-tested therapeutic tradition that survived centuries and cultural differences.

The idea behind crystal healing today is to use crystals to help you bring back your inner balance, get rid of stress, and boost your energy levels.

How do Crystals Work?

As living beings possessing their own energy, crystals have the power to influence your energy balance and level of health. Crystals radiate their own vibrations that can positively affect your vibrations. Each crystal carries its own unique characteristics and while some emit energy-lifting vibrations, others can produce a soothing effect. Therefore, it's important to learn to distinguish the different types of crystals and their uses. Doing so will aid you in using and balancing your combination of crystals to fit your present needs.

Everything in this world is made up of energy. That includes you, too. Your entire being is energy, which manifests in various patterns and densities. If you study your own anatomy and note how the various systems work together, you'll agree that it is but a replica of the ecosystem. The same is true with all living beings on this earth. Your state of health depends entirely on whether these energy patterns can preserve their perfect balance. A disruption in the pattern brings about illness.

The great news is everything in this universe was created with the gift to heal, if not others, then at least itself. Your lifestyle and various internal and external factors continuously interrupt your body's delicate balance (ex. lack of sleep, too much work, and exposure to daily stressors). Still, it's possible to restore the harmony by drawing energy from something which possesses innate balance. This is where healing crystals come in. Simply put, the secret is in the structure. It's because of their natural makeup that crystals are so effective in stabilizing one's emotions, psyche and physical body systems.

In healing, crystals are used as vibratory tools. Humans are such emotional beings that we are also extremely mutable. Plainly put, it's easy to go out of tune. A quartz plate, on the other hand, possesses its own resonant frequency and maintains it. Each time a current passes through a quartz plate, the current will oscillate according to the crystal's resonant frequency. Think of how great it would be if you allow that kind of stability to rub off on you.

But can it? Can the stable quality of crystals really rub off on me?

Imagine two singers. One has a weak voice. The other has a loud voice. Put them together and ask them to sing side by side. The singer with a weak voice also ends up with a stronger and more resonant voice. That's because each time you bring together two objects with the same frequency, the one who possesses the weaker frequency will instantly bring itself into line with the object with the more powerful frequency. In chronobiology, this is called entrainment. Thus, when you place the *right* crystal in close proximity to your body, it will keep your body in tune, so to speak.

How Effective is Crystal Healing?

The effectiveness of crystal healing depends on several factors such as whether you were using the right crystal, whether your crystal was properly cleansed, etc. But more importantly, the success of crystal healing will depend hugely on your receptiveness.

Chapter 4: Selecting Your Crystals

While picking crystals for your very own use and beginning, ensure you have at any rate two of every primary color you will work with. This incorporates red, orange, yellow, green, blue, purple, pink, white, clear, and black. Colors of the crystals are related to our chakra focuses and can likewise compare to a portion of the afflictions. It is a great idea to have a wide assortment of crystals and crystal stones to have close by when working.

My undisputed top choices to keep close by are: Hematite, Peridot, Rhodonite, Bloodstone, Topaz, Turquoise, Red Jasper, Rose Quartz, Carnelian, Amber, Tiger's Eye, Malachite, Moss Agate, Turquoise, Aquamarine, Moonstone, Smoky Quartz, Onyx, Lapis Lazuli, Amethyst, Fluorite, Clear Quartz,, and Black Tourmaline.

There are numerous crystals and crystal stones out there, so do whatever it takes not to get overpowered and befuddled picking or picking which ones are directly for you or be concerned if you didn't get the correct ones. The best manual for picking your own crystals is to pursue your instinct. Your instinct will never guide you wrong if you hear it out. At times it very well may be challenging to comprehend if you have not worked with following your "gut" senses previously, yet hear them out when working with crystals.

At the point when you first go out to pick your new crystals, ensure you are in a positive and upbeat state of mind. You would prefer not to attract negative fiery sentiments, so put on some glad music in the vehicle and consider something that you appreciate while you are headed to the crystal shop.

When you arrive, proceed to begin glancing around to perceive what grabs your attention first. Get the crystal and check whether it feels right to you. If it does, search for additional to add to your very own crystal healing pack. If it does not, put it down and move to another!

There is no set in stone answer, however crossbeam what resounds inside you!

Simply recall that your crystals will pick you the same amount as you pick them!

If you feel any sensations, for example, shivering, or quietness, then that crystal is a decent counterpart for what you require it for. In any case, don't surrender if you don't feel anything when you touch a crystal. This doesn't mean it won't work for you, and it just means it should be used alternately, for example, worn or set on the proper chakra.

Picking crystals shouldn't be excessively convoluted, however. Try not to be hesitant to pick a crystal since it is a pretty color and grabs your attention. There is an explanation these crystals attract your eye to them, and if they do, then these are crystals you ought to have.

To assist you with beginning gathering your crystals, here are six that you ought to have in your assortment:

Clear Quartz

This crystal is viewed as an all-inclusive crystal for healing. It is an unquestionable requirement has for anybody, particularly that only starting to dig into the universe of crystal healing. Not exclusively does this crystal lift the energy of the wearer, it additionally secures against the adverse energies of different people and can help your immune system. Clear Quartz can be used to clean various crystals, and it should be washed down consistently. You can do this by holding it under running water and putting it in the sun for a couple of hours.

Citrine

Commonly found in yellow or champagne color ranges, Citrine has creative and chipper energy. This makes it a perfect crystal to wear or use when your disposition is maybe low, or you need assistance with imagination. This crystal is likewise used to help whatever worries success and accounts. It is otherwise called a crystal of karma and certainty. Some even consider it the 'shipper's stone' because of its capacity to pull in business and cash. In contrast to the clear quartz, Citrine shouldn't be heald each week, however ought to be purified on occasion by holding it under running water.

Green Aventurine

Aventurine is a kind of quartz that arrives in an assortment of hues, yet the green tones are prescribed for using as healing crystals. Green Aventurine is a crystal that symbolizes wellbeing and essentialness. It is this way valuable for anything to do with certainty, welfare, companions, money, and development.

Rose Quartz

Viewed as the widespread crystal of adoration, yet it's not only for pulling in affection and sentiment. Rose Quartz likewise heals and advance self-acknowledgment and self-esteem to the client. It accomplishes this by reinforcing and clearing the heart chakra. It expels past damages and encounters from the heart, enabling it to be available to adore. This quartz has a very quieting impact and feeling for some, who hold or wear it. To wash down rose quartz, hold it under running water, then lay it close to clear quartz to energize its energy.

Amethyst

Maybe the most prominent crystal of all, regardless of whether for healing or just due to its vibe, amethyst can be found in a full scope of violet and purple tints. Amethyst is used for decontaminating air and in-depth insurance, just as making harmony between the psychological, passionate, and physical bodies. Regularly used in contemplation, amethyst is known to help increase instinct. Its quieting capacities can help with physical sicknesses, for example, migraines and an assortment of addictions. It ought to be heald in a similar way as the rose quartz, yet don't leave it in the daylight as the color can change whenever uncovered for a long time.

Black Tourmaline

This specific crystal is broadly recognized as an establishing stone and is a defender from negative energy, including that from electronic gadgets. At the point when it is worn, it repulses the antagonistic energy away from the individual wearing the crystal. It is additionally valuable to use if you are feeling confounded, perplexed, or absent-minded. In the same way as other different crystals, it can likewise be washed down by holding it underneath running water then laying in the daylight to energize.

Chapter 5: What, Exactly, Is Chakra?

First things first: what is the literal meaning of chakra? I'm borrowing that leaf of procedure from teachers because they tell us the best way to understand something is to move from the known to the mysterious. So, by that count, you need, from the onset, to understand that chakra literally means **wheel** or even **disk**; and that notion has its origin in Sanskrit.

That is San – what? Yes – Sanskrit; the official language of Uttarakhand, a state in India. And that is not all. In Hinduism, Jainism and also Buddhism, Sanskrit is the liturgical and philosophical language.

Basically, in the Indian way of thinking, chakras are points where spiritual power converges within the human body. In fact, in Ayurveda, yoga and also meditation, chakra actually refers to the wheels that circulate energy in currents through your body. So, generally speaking, chakra has everything to do with the spiritual energy working best within your physical body to give you harmony and well-being. And while chakra is the particular point of energy convergence, the energy itself is referred to as **Prana**, which essentially means breath.

But why do we need to know about chakras?

See: consideringthatchakras are responsibleforyour well-being irrespective of whether you are rich or poor, are they then not very important to you? You need to appreciate that these chakras are the ones that let that important universal energy flow through your body systematically, thus making you feel alive, well and optimistic about life. For that reason, it is important that they remain open to facilitate that healthy flow of energy.

What can jeopardize the good working of a chakra?

Naturally, chakras are meant to remain open. But we jeopardize that when we do things that cause their blockage. For instance, when you get upset and you do not deal with the cause of your anger, you remain tense, and you, effectively, block the chakra concerned.

So chakras do not work the same?

No, chakras do not play the same role in the body. Granted, they all facilitate smooth and harmonious flow of energy in your body, but each chakra has its specific role. Have in mind that you have seven chakras, and they all need to be balanced lest you fall ill or feel uncomfortable. That balancing act encompasses your body, your mind and your soul. If one of those elements is out of balance, there is no way you will be fine. You may feel depressed, unsettled, or just lacking in enthusiasm.

To understand how different chakras operate, you need to know that they are categorized distinctly: matter related chakras; spirit related chakras; and the chakra that is the link between the matter and spirit chakras.

Matter related chakras

Chakra One

This is called Muladhara. It is the chakra that makes you feel like a lion; knowing no fear wherever you are and in whatever you are doing. It makes you have a sense of security. This chakra is in charge of stability; security; and your other fundamental needs.

Any idea where this 1*st* chakra is situated? Well – go right to the area of your spine and count from up – one; two; and three. Those three vertebrae are part of the first chakra. Besides those vertebrae, there is the bladder and the colon. So, you will only feel safe and bold when the chakra covering this particular zone is open, enabling free flow of energy through these organs.

Chakra Two

This particular chakra is referred to as Svadhisthana. It is the chakra to take care of if you want your creative sense to remain alert and active; and your sensuality too.

The location of the 2nd chakra…?

Right on yourlower body: between the navel and the pubic bone. So when you are feeling creative about things, whether in your job, your hobby or even in relationships, revel in the fact that your chakra Number 2 is open. In fact, you need to make a conscious effort to keep that area in good shape.

Chakra Three

This is the chakra known as Manipura. It is the one in charge of our inner most power; that which makes you appreciate things with clarity and you are selfassured. With this chakra working well, you make intelligent decisions with confidence and you feel blissful.

Area of occupation of Chakra 3...?

Right aboveyour navel but below your breastbone is where your third chakra resides. If you want to feel in charge of things, that is the area of your body to take care of.

The spirit related chakras

Chakra Five

This fifth chakra is referred to as Vishuddha. It facilitates your effective flow of your speech, and it enables and encourages you to say only that which is true.

Physical location of Chakra 5...?

This chakra is found around your throat; encompassing your neck; your thyroid and also parathyroid glands; your jaw; your mouth; and tongue as well. As is evident, all these organs are very much part of your speech formulation. As such, as thewords form and also other sounds of speech, Vishuddha, this fifth chakra, sees to their quality and integrity.

Chakra Six

This chakra is known as Ajna. It gives you that intuitive sense. When you feel right about something even without having evaluated it deeply, or alternatively, you feel hesitant about something with no facts to support your hesitation, it is this sixth chakra at play, communicating to you and helping you make a fitting decision.

Where is this 6th chakra situated?

Notsurprisingly, Ajna, the sixth chakra, is located some place in your head – that is, right between your eyebrows. So if you take care of this area and ensure this chakra is allowing free flow of energy, you will get warnings about looming danger or a boost of encouragement to move ahead with things that are bound to benefit you immensely. This is, definitely, beneficial to your being, whether you are alone or amongst other people.

Chakra Seven

This seventh chakra is called Sahaswara. It is the chakra that enables you to be in touch with yourself at the deepest level. It also enables you to be in touch with the divine power. Generally, this chakra enables a healthy spiritual connection between you and other people and also with the divine power.

Where is the 7*th* chakra located?

This chakra thathelps us understand where we stand spiritually is situated where the crown of the head is.

The chakra linking the spirit related and matter related chakras

Chakra Four

This 4*th* chakra is known as Anahata. It is the chakra that ensures a harmonious connection between the other two groups of chakras: those that are spirit related and those that are matter related. Though this chakra is a link between the lower and the upper chakras, this 4*th* chakra is essentially spirit-oriented; also being the smooth link between your body and the set of intangibles that are your mind; your emotions; and your spirit.

Physical location of the 4*th* chakra…?

This is the heart. Anahata, the 4*th* chakra, resides in your heart. Andsowhenyourheart is healthy in allrespects, there is a sense of well-beingthatyou sense, both at physical and spiritual level.

One thing you need to understand is that, generally, when your chakras of the physical body work well, your spiritual ones work relatively well too. So what we need to learn is how to keep the chakras open and enable harmonious working of the body functions at all levels. In subsequent chapters, therefore, you are going to see how to open up your chakras to enable that free flow of spiritual energy, a process that leads to you leading a peaceful life of optimism and happiness.

Chapter 6: The Power Of Crystal

Crystals have consistently been viewed as a wellspring of power—and as a blessing from the divine beings. Noteworthy, regardless of their size, gems hold an atmosphere of secret, and authority. From ancient times to the present, gemstones have symbolized riches and been agreed to remarkable properties. The antiquated writings that enlighten us so much regarding the power of stones had their starting points in the Stone Age where innovation originated from stones. Since that time, we have kept on tackling their mystical power.

In 1714, M. B. Valentine's Museum Muserum imagined an aircraft structured five years sooner by a Brazilian minister; the art was to be powered by Agate and iron that, when warmed in the sun, would get attractive. Abnormal as this may appear, our present-day innovation couldn't exist without crystals; they power PCs and careful apparatuses, coat car motors, and spaceships— crystals give the essential structure squares of science and craftsmanship.

The people of yore acknowledged crystals for healing power. The Greek scholar Theophrastus and Roman geographer Pliny passed these cures on (Even though Pliny criticized some as bogus cases). The Babylonians credited humanity's fate on the impact of valuable stones. Our predecessors accepted that the Earth was encompassed by crystal circles where divine beings,stars, and planets abided. Initially, a crystal's color or constitution or its planetary association demonstrated its adequacy for explicit conditions. Shockingly, interpretation troubles frequently make it difficult to learn precisely which stone first messages alluded to; however, a few references are crystal clear.

Formats of Light

Every crystal has its very own remarkable energy signature. These "Layouts of light" are encoded with all as you have to initiate your very own power. The key is to discover a crystal that is sensitive to your very own energy, or that raises your vigorous reverberation to guarantee prosperity and grow your cognizance.

The Power of Gems

Not just showy gemstones hold power. Since vestige, crystals of numerous types have filled in as defensive ornaments. Humble stones, for example, Flint, were supernatural transporters for the spirit, for otherworldly activities, or for shamans to use on their extraordinary voyages. Numerous stones delivered brilliant starts or could be super-warmed into surges of gold, silver, copper, and different valuable metals. Just as enchanted were the sky shakes that tumbled to Earth, carrying with them, iron to produce instruments and make weapons.

Egyptologist Wallis Budge clarified, "Each stone had a kind of living character, which could encounter infection, and ailment, and could get old.

Furthermore, powerless and even bite the dust." However, in Egyptian medicine, stones could likewise recuperate. The Greek scholar Plato accepted stones were living creatures, delivered by a maturation procedure instigated by "A nurturing knowledge dropping from the stars." According to numerous legends, crystals cemented from ice, a view strengthened by the air pockets of water some of the time found inside a crystal.

The fifth-century Roman artist Claudian discloses to us that:

At the point when the Alpine ice, ice-hardened into stone

First overcame the sun, and as a gemstone,

Not all its substance could the gem accept some noticeable drops still lingered in its belly.

HOW CRYSTALS FORM

Crystals are, generally, made by the Earth's marvelous power.

Bubbled, packed, and abraded, some were conceived of volcanoes, icy masses, quakes, and gigantic weight; others trickled into being without really trying, gas air pockets, and nature's gentler powers.

A few supposed crystals don't have a crystalline structure. Golden, for occurrence, is fossilized tree sap, and volcanic Obsidian framed so quick it didn't have the opportunity to crystallize— how a crystal structure influences how its power functions. Those that became gradually will, in general, emanate their power tenderly; those that were on a quickened way of development shoot their power out to the world. Incomprehensibly, the absolute most youthful land stones have the most elevated vibrations, and the most prominent power to change our reality.

The Power of Color

The people of the old first recorded the power of color. It turned into a necessary some portion of the mysterious healing procedures by which lopsided characteristics were amended, and concordance reestablished. In 1878, Edwin D. Babbitt recommended color had healing properties that could be applied in healing. His method of reasoning may clarify the power behind thoughtful enchantment and why specific colors customarily were used to treat specific maladies. In Babbitt's "Beam" framework, red draws in iron, zinc, Strontium; yellow sodium, phosphorous, and carbon, etc. These minerals are required for the right working of the body. His Chroma therapy was Complex, and introduction to the colored beams should have been painstakingly aligned.

Crystal laborers, however, mostly use crystals of the proper color based on the antiquated correspondences.

• Pink and peach stones mend passionate, awkward nature and tenderly stimulate your system.

• Red gems invigorate all the more powerfully and reverberate with the regenerative framework. Red additionally helps blood-related and provocative conditions.

• Orange is a psychological and innovative energizer, invigorating individual power and reverberating with the Leydig organ over the testicles, a seat of kundalini power.

- Yellow and gold stones are mental and sensory system triggers; they reverberate with synapses, the adrenal organs, and digestion tracts to balance your brain and feelings.

Green is quieting and connected with the heart, eyes, and thymus organ.

- Blue-green resounds with the unobtrusive degrees of being and opens supernatural capacities.
- Blue reverberates with the throat and thyroid organ and has a tonic impact.
- Indigo has enchanted characteristics; it resounds with the pineal organ, yet additionally impacts mental healing.
- Violet and purple stones reverberate with the pituitary, directing digestion and, recovering the body— they additionally open you to higher mindfulness.
- Black and dark-colored stones detoxify and ground energy, securing the body from hurt.
- Combination stones synergize the impacts of the colors and constituents.

The Power of Magic

For thrice seven days, the active wizard fled the shower's refreshment and his associate's bed. For thrice seven days, a grave quick kept up. At that point in the living wellspring, the gem leaves.

As to a divine being, he forfeits brings and, intense spells in spiritualist mumbles sings. Till moved by extraordinary petition and powerful charms, a living soul, the farsighted substance warms.

At that point in his grasp, he bears the thing divine, where encouraged lights in his unadulterated manor sparkle. Also, as her newborn child, a mother holds, so in her arms, the charm he overlaps. Also, thou, if thou wouldst hear the spiritualist voice, hence do, furthermore, in the wondrous thing celebrate. The Lithia Crystals have consistently been credited with having supernatural power, as the above citation from a third-century B.C.E. stone book appears. It likewise depicts the wonderment and reverence with which they were taken care of. Enchantment isn't pure superstition—it is the establishment for the trial sciences that the advanced world is qualities so exceptionally of. Without enchantment, we would not have medicine, stargazing, writing and show, science, arithmetic, music, folklore, and maybe indeed, even religion itself. Mysterious formulae establish the absolute most seasoned works, and it could be contended that the letter set—also the chronicle of information itself—is a type of enchantment. Enchantment isn't only a lot of practices and convictions; it is a method for taking a gander at the world. The view that the natural world was enlivening, bursting at the seams with otherworldly powers interpenetrating the substance of the physical and the mystical domains administered old life, and passing. Crystal laborers today still collaborate with the vivify powers, the living creatures, inside crystals.

The word enchantment originates from magi, the savvy people of Persia and Babylon, yet has its foundations in the Sumerian word image signifying "profound" or "significant." Magic was a method for controlling the regular world and drawing in support of the divine beings, yet besides, as anthropologist Robert Ranulph Marett lets us know, "A higher plane of experience . . . in which profound enlargement is valued for the good of its own."

Such vast numbers of new crystals are entering the market today that it very well may be trying to keep up or to know which ones will be beneficial.

Each is ascribed an extraordinary power that summarizes its overall impact, yet I offer a more great depiction of its healing and transformational properties too. You'll discover crystals for adoration, wellbeing, insurance, bounty, life span, equity, and the sky is the limit from there.

Not all crystals suit everybody, so my determination offers options and new conceivable outcomes to resound with your one of a kind energy field. I additionally disclose how to tackle every crystal's power. When you become acclimated with working with crystals, you can apply these strategies to your different crystals.

The chakra graph with information can additionally help you in working with stones. A glossary beginning on clarifies terms with which you might be new. Guidelines for picking fitting crystals, just as cleaning, actuating, and keeping up their powers

High-Vibration Crystals

A few crystals, for example, Selenite and Danburite, effectively had a light, high vibration that actuates the higher chakras. In any case, new finds of Danburite and others surely understood crystals that have a higher-vibration of the essential power have become accessible. For instance, regular Golden Danburite (Agni Gold™) and the chemicalized Aqua Aura Danburite have the fundamental properties of the essential Danburite crystal, yet raise these to another measurement.

Instructions to Find the Right Crystal for You

Look for not to quantify the material, yet consider instead the power which reason has and negligible substance, not Manilius (Roman soothsayer)

Finding the correct stone for you is simply the way to adjusting to crystal power. Be that as it may, what would be the best next step? Imagine a scenario where you have no clue which crystal is directly for you?

Use your own mystical power of fascination! Put out the focused idea: "I find precisely the correct crystal for me, presently. This is the crystal for you. You may, as of now, have the right stone in your assortment. Any place you discover your crystal, ensure you sanitize and empower it before use. While picking a crystal, recollect the greatest and flashiest isn't the best for your motivation. The Roman artist Claudian offered a saying savvy crystal laborer still use today:

Pass not the undefined chunk of crystal or see the cold mass with the reckless eye.

This unpleasant and unformed stone, without an effortlessness,

Middle rarest fortunes hold the chiefest spot.

It isn't the outward magnificence of a crystal that shows its power, but instead what it accomplishes for you. A flat piece of crude stone might be more potent than a faceted gemstone, regardless of how alluring the last might be.

Crystal Attunement

Take some moments to adjust to a crystal. Hold a cleaned crystal in your hands and feel its vibrations emanating into your being. If they are your own, you will contact quiet, tranquil, and potentially extended. On the off chance that you feel awkward, pick another stone—the one you are holding probably won't be directly for you right now, or may show you have internal work to do.

The Power of Shape

Crystals usually have inside and outside geometric shapes, which shape how energy courses through them. Be that as it may, numerous crystals are falsely molded remotely to upgrade their power stream. Knowing how the outside shape improves the power encourages you to select the correct crystal for your motivation.

Take Amethyst, for instance. You'll discover Amethyst in cakelike geodes, single points, clusters, beds, balls, and palm stones. All convey Amethyst's fundamental significant serenity; however, how that power emanates differs as indicated by the stone's shape.

GEODE

The cave-like the inside of a geode gathers, enhances, and stores crystal power, and afterward, delicately emanates it out to the earth. It gives insurance, makes wealth, and supports profound development.

POINT

Points, including wands, center crystal power into a solitary concentrated bar—at the point when you place the position toward your body, it channels its power into your body. Point the end out, and it draws off negative energy.

Ghost

Ghost crystals are set down in layers, frequently pyramidal fit as a fiddle, inside another sort of crystal. Holding the memory of the spirit's adventure, they separate old examples of conduct, or can be climbed like a stepping stool to higher cognizance.

CLUSTER

Clusters are a gathering of points emanating out in various ways. The shaft energy into the encompassing climate, yet can likewise be empowered to draw off

BED

A bed has numerous little crystals spread over a grid base— this gives a consistent wellspring of crystal power, similar to a battery does. Beds are especially useful at the point when you need eternal crystal power.

BALL

Balls are misleadingly formed from a more significant part of crystal; they emanate power in all bearings in equivalent measure. Balls give a concentration to powers, for example, knowledge, or then again instinct. Customarily, crystal balls were used to see forward or, in reverse in time, a training known as scrying.

PALM STONE

Level and adjusted, palm stones are material tokens of crystal power. Holding one alleviates the brain, so that your central goal can make what you want.

MANIFESTATION

This crystal has a littler crystal encased inside the fundamental one. As its name recommends, it conveys the power of appearance—particularly of wealth—yet can be the outfit to any crystal power.

Keeping up Crystal Power

Crystals must be refined and actuated to breathe life into their power, and they must be kept rinsed to keep up that power. It is nothing more than trouble purchasing a crystal, placing it in your pocket, and anticipating that it should work marvels except if you've asked it to. As an initial step, like Shakespeare, who knew about the obscure power of stones, trains in Henry V, "Go, clear thy crystals?" Once you've refined your crystal, its power can be devoted to your most elevated high.

Approach your crystals with deference and work with them in an association. They will reimburse you with long stretches of committed assistance. Treat them gravely or misuse them, and their power may betray you— they are mysterious and conscious creatures.

RIGHT USE OF POWER

Crystals work by helping out you to center and show your goal.

Be clear concerning why you are working with the crystal and guarantee that you are working for the most elevated great. Misuse of crystal power will unavoidably bounce back.

Like humans, crystals can get depleted, so re-empowering them routinely is a reasonable safeguard. As crystals quickly draw off energy from their environment, they need filtering at visit interims.

PURIFYING YOUR CRYSTALS

Crystals get energy from any individual who handles them and from the condition, so they need purging when use. Refine a crystal by holding it under running water— insofar as the crystal won't break down or part. At that point, put it in the sun or evening glow to reenergize it. You can likewise smirch a crystal with incense smoke, place it in candlelight, or leave it medium-term in uncooked dark colored rice.

INITIATING THE POWER OF YOUR CRYSTAL

To initiate your crystal's power, grasp the cleaned crystal, concentrate your expectation and consideration on it, and state:

"I commit this crystal to the most elevated great of all furthermore, ask that its power be actuated presently to work inconsistency with my own will, and focused aim."

On the off chance that you have a particular reason, add that to your devotion. To deactivate the crystal, rinse it and afterward hold the crystal as you state:

"I appreciate this crystal for its energy, which is never again required at this time. I ask that its power be shut until reactivated."

Put the crystal in the sun to energize it, and afterward place it in a pack, box, or a cabinet until it is required once more.

If you are placing crystals in a network, format for cleaning, or making safe space, sign up the shape either by contacting each stone with a crystal wand or by utilizing the power of your brain to picture lines of light associating the stones and making the shape.

Utilizing Crystal Power

After you have approved your crystal, you can dress with it day by day, ideally in contact with your skin. Or then again, place it on your body or in your condition to emanate out or draw on the power as proper. A bit of Black Tourmaline or Golden, for example, set in each edge of your home, conjures the power of assurance and energy screening, protecting you, or on the other hand, you can use your crystal for healing or grow your awareness.

Probably the most straightforward approach to take advantage of a crystal's healing power is to put the crystal over a proper chakra or organ for fifteen minutes to rebalance the energy focus. Regular purging and reenergizing of your chakras (the body's clairvoyant insusceptible framework) keep up your energy at ideal levels and animates your power.

Chapter 7: The Use Of Crystals

Using crystal bracelet is one good way to make excellent use of this wonderful group of crystals. There are so many possibilities that you will surely be able to get a piece that suits your needs. Wearing a beautiful piece of quartz jewelry like the smoky quartz crystal pendant shown below is a good choice to wear as a jewel.

Other varieties of quartz that have excellent metaphysical properties that make them beneficial to maintain in your body include pink quartz crystal, Prasiolite also known as green amethyst crystals, yellow Citrine crystals and purple amethyst crystals.

The use of quartz crystals allows you to continually use the protective and grounding energies they emit. A beautiful bracelet, pendant or natural quartz crystal necklace has a powerful energy. The smoky quartz crystals are a very useful quartz crystal to use. Using one of these natural crystals, be it a pendant, a ring or another jewel, keeps them within their aura and can create a healing effect of quartz crystal. Since the earth naturally irradiates smoky quartz, it can be useful to help cancer patients undergo radiation treatment. The necklaces or pendants of smoky quartz or tourmaline Quartz are powerful aids for psychic protection and to protect you from negativity and for the spiritual base, they are excellent assets.

If the jewelry is too expensive for you, you can use a small stone from any of the quartz crystals by keeping it in your pocket during the day. While they are within your aura, their energy will benefit you. Remember to perform one of the cleaning processes of your crystals regularly. Cleaning quartz crystals is much easier than cleaning other crystals, so be sure to do it regularly to keep your vibration high. This includes cleaning your crystal jewelry.

How will Healing with Crystals Help You?

Healing with quartz crystals can promote the release of negativity and stimulate positive thoughts and feelings. There is a wide assortment of quartz varieties that you can choose to try. The quartz amplification property will send the energy of any variety of crystal you have chosen to the space where you are.

It is even possible to buy quartz that has been carved in the form of crystal skulls. To heal on a spiritual level, they are especially powerful. Quartz crystal is also used to make glass bowls, pendulums and crystal wands used for healing. Natural Lemurian crystal wands are also wonderful tools for healing. Think of using quartz crystal if you have not already done so. It is easy to get and easy to buy. You will be happily surprised at how good the amethyst crystals or a piece of rose quartz crystal feels in your room.

Still thinking Whether to Heal with Crystals?

Crystal therapy is an ancient art, which is generally referred to as healing stones. It is an alternative medicine technique and those who practice it believe that crystals and stones can cure ailments and other diseases. Crystal therapy was conceived by ancient civilizations to balance the chakras and to transform the energy properties of the body, resulting in a clean energy field. This natural form of healing is often used today to create relaxation and relieve stress.

Chapter 8: Colors And Chakras

The Chakra System

It is important when exploring crystals and their powers to understand the chakra system. Many crystals embody a specific energy associated with a specific chakra, therefore learning about the chakras can help you access the metaphysical properties of crystals and bring greater self-development into life. Chakras are essentially portals of energy linking to our physical bodies. They connect through the ether- where illness, disease, and distortion originate- and where healing can take place to influence all aspects of life. Emotions, detrimental thought patterns, blocks and issues in sexual, spiritual, or physical health can all be overcome through chakra work. Crystals and consciousness are deeply linked. Chakra comes from ancient Sanskrit and literally means energy wheel, or energy portal. Each chakra corresponds with a physical body part, organ or area. There are seven major energetic centers within each level of the aura, joined together at intervals along the spine. They are constantly moving, absorbing currents of energy; the chakras are an essential part of our bio-energy system. A free flow of life-giving energy is vital to the health and well-being of the individual. The electro-magnetic energy circulating around the body stimulates various glands, thus maintaining hormonal balance and affecting our whole metabolism.

The chakras enable us to gather, process and release energy from the earth and from the atmosphere around us. They feed the life-force into our endocrine system, which in turn stimulates and regulates our hormonal balance. So, although the chakra system exists in the etheric body, it has close connection and interrelates with the physical body. The chakra conducts and filters a constant flow of energy through us. Crystals can help maintain this balanced flow. All life forms have chakra centers, and these act as conductors of energy. It is believed that the mineral kingdom has one chakra, the animal kingdom has three or four, and it is only in man that we have three transpersonal centers linking us and allowing us to communicate with the divine world. There are seven main chakras and twenty-one minor ones. It is a good idea to learn the positions of the minor chakras as well as the major ones, for crystals or gemstones can be very effective when laid on these places. The major chakras are found at the base of the spine, the sacral center, the solar plexus, the heart, the throat, the brow or third eye and the crown. Sometimes an eighth chakra is included, and this is situated at the thymus gland, which is located above the heart and below the throat centers. We are coming to realize that the thymus chakra is of great importance at this time, as it appears to affect our immune system. Here we explore the **7** main chakras in more detail, with a light examination of the 8th; the thymus gland.

The Root Chakra

Introduction: THE BASE CENTRE
Color: **Red**
Element: Earth energy

The base center relates to the life-force energy and is the spirit of life. The color red gives us physical strength and vitality. It is a stimulant and has heating qualities and controls the creative, procreative and restorative functions of the body. You can use red where there is an inability to accept life's responsibilities and if someone tends to be too dominant, dogmatic and pushy.

The root chakra is also known as the Muladhara chakra in Sanskrit (mula means root). It is essentially the foundation where kundalini energy, or shakti, arises. Kundalini energy is also known as serpent power and relates to sexuality, vitality, health, and psychic abilities. To many, sexual energy and psychic energy are one and the same, hence why many schools of thought equate tantric sex as the highest form of sexual expression and union. Physically, the root chakra is located just below the genitalia and any blockages here can lead to problems in energy flow up the spine through the other chakras. Crystals which relate to the root are usually red, brown, and 'earthy' in color. It is important to make sure you have a strong and healthy root and work with crystals which can help. Disruptions in this chakra can lead to ill health and interferences in sexual vitality, energy and passion for life, creative expression, emotional connection and maturity, confidence and self-empowerment issues, expression, communication, feelings of love, empathy and kindness, and the ability to perceive subtle energy and be open to new ways of seeing.

Crystals for the root chakra: Obsidian, Black Onyx, Hematite, Black Tourmaline, Smoky Quartz, Red Jasper, Bloodstone, Ruby and Garnet.

The Sacral Chakra

Introduction: THE SACRAL CENTRE

Color: **Orange**

Element: **Water energy** relating to the emotions

The sacral center relates to the spirit of health. Orange energizes the adrenals and kidneys energizing the body physically, nourishing it by absorbing nutrients from food. The sacral chakra corresponds to the spleen from where stems our ability to experience joy. The sacral chakra is the center of the emotional body, and orange can stimulate a loving warm contact with others. This center governs our sexuality and this energy can be channeled into creative and artistic development. Use orange for the fearful and timid, orange helps shyness and lack of interest in life.

The sacral chakra is the second chakra and relates to emotions, sexual memories, and creativity. Working with crystals which are orange are particularly effective for the sacral as this color induces feelings of warmth, intimacy, and connection. A healthy sacral chakra is symbolized by emotional health, wisdom and maturity, positive sexual memories and feelings towards sex and intimacy, and a profound level of sexual and shadow acceptance. The sacral is also strongly associated with creativity and the ability to be able to express oneself creatively. Blockages, however, can manifest as disorders including, but not exclusive to, addictions, sexual expressions, inauthenticity, creative blocks, jealousies, envies and resentments, fears and anxieties, wounds, traumas and feelings of guilt, and shame or victimhood. Luckily, there are crystals which can help with all of these.

Crystals for the Sacral Chakra: Carnelian, Coral, Orange Jasper, Moonstone, Pearl, and Citrine.

The Solar Plexus Chakra

Introduction: THE SOLAR-PLEXUS

Color: **Yellow**

Element: **Fire energy** relating to the seat of Power

This chakra relates to the autonomic nervous system, pancreas and liver. Yellow has a stimulating effect on the nerves. It is good for coordination and orientation. It aids digestion and purifies the whole system and is especially good for the skin. Yellow links to the mental and intellectual faculties and encourages warmheartedness. Yellow dispels envy, jealousy and fear. It counteracts feelings of lack of power or obsessional behavior.

The third chakra, your solar plexus, is just above your navel region and can be effectively healed through crystals which are yellow or gold. In Sanskrit, it is known as the Manipura chakra and literally translates as the dwelling place of the jewel (gem/jewel: mani, dwelling place: pura). This is understandable when we look at the energy and symbolism of the solar plexus chakra. Confidence, self-empowerment, will, ego, action, expression, and self-sovereignty all come under the solar plexus, as does self-esteem and self-worth, ambitions, dreams and aspirations. It is essentially your will and has strong links to the sun. Crystals which are specifically for the sacral are usually to enhance confidence, self-esteem, bring empowerment, and steer you onto new directions in alignment with goals, dreams, and aspirations. They can also help develop a healthy ego if you are lacking in individuality or suffer from self-sacrifice, excessive people-pleasing or victimhood, martyrdom and savior complexes.

Crystals for the Solar Plexus: Tigers Eye, Citrine, Topaz, Yellow Fluorite, Agate, Amber, Peacock Ore, Pyrite and Peridot.

The Heart Chakra

Introduction: THE HEART

Color: **Green**

Element: **Air/earth energy** relating to unconditional love.

The heart chakra is linked to our true soul emotions and our ability to give and receive unconditional love. Green links to the heart center and affects the physical heart and blood circulation. Green is found in the center of the spectrum. It is neither a cool nor a warm color and is therefore entirely neutral. Green can be used in healing to compliment any of the other colors. It harmonizes, its energy restoring balance and bringing peace. When the heart chakra is open it brings with it understanding, sympathy and co-operation with others and with nature. Green is the color of evolution and we have to learn to trust the process of life. Pink is also related to the heart, for pink symbolizes divine love. Give treatments using pink and green stones where there is insecurity and a needing to be loved and protected. Green and pink is also good for feelings that life is unfair, unjust and a victim mentality.

The heart or anahata chakra (Sanskrit) is the center. It is the chakra linking lower self and higher self; the genitalia, sexual organs, bodily functions and desires, and the upper energy centers. In this sense, it relates to compassion, empathy, understanding for others, and unconditional love. People with a strong heart chakra usually have a real love for the natural world and are drawn towards helping others in some way, or at least exhibit frequent and genuine displays of kindness, generosity, and affection. Issues or disruptions in the heart chakra can lead to greed, envy, vindictiveness, jealousy, anger, rage, codependency, and a lack of self-love. Other characteristics common when there is a disruption of energy in the heart chakra include judgment, possessiveness, emotional manipulation, coldness, hatred, spite, and the inability to express love. Crystals specifically for the heart chakra can help to alleviate these problems and also bring lots of positive qualities and characteristics (these will be explored in Chapter 5).

Crystals for the Heart Chakra: Emerald, Jade, Diamond, Malachite, Tree Moss Agate, Aventurine, Ruby, Rhodonite, Green Agate, Kunzite, and Rose Quartz.

The Thymus (8th chakra)

Introduction: THE THYMUS (the existence of this chakra is not universally accepted)

Color: **Turquoise**

Element: Water energy

Some people believe that there is a chakra that exists in between the heart chakra and the throat chakra. This chakra is a very powerful energy channel that links you to the earth and to the heavens. Uniting with this chakra brings about great awareness to your emotional and spiritual planes. The thymus gland helps produce antibodies, which protect our immune system.

Turquoise energy encourages well-adjustment and the capability of interacting with people socially. It brings freshness of ideas helping change negative thinking and purity of thought. Use turquoise for confusion, turmoil, and an inability to move through your own boundaries and limitations. It helps dispel destructive thought forms, i.e. I can't do it, I'm no good, and I am ugly. etc.

Stones: Cleanse, purify and balance. Turquoise, Chrysoprase.

The Throat Chakra

Introduction: THE THROAT

Color: **Blue**

Element: Ether, and Air energy

Blue controls the metabolic rate of the thyroid and parathyroid glands, so balancing the bodies' equilibrium. It is cooling and soothing to the mind and affects our ability to express ourselves vocally. This means it helps us communicate our inner feelings and needs to others. Use blue power where there is a difficulty in motivation and difficulty in expressing yourself and also if you are involved in things which have little to do with everyday life. Related stones cleanse and clear the etheric body.

The throat chakra relates to all aspects of communication. Song, speech, musical expression, written communication, writing, and expression of feelings and emotions all come under this chakra realm. If there is a blockage in the throat chakra it will have a profound effect on all levels of being. This is because suppression of expression links intrinsically to emotions, feelings, and beliefs. If we feel we are not able to speak our truth, stand in our wisdom, or express ourselves in any way, this will only lead to disruptions in energy flow. Over time these minor blockages accumulate to form severe problems, mainly in the sacral and third eye chakra. This is due to the connection between emotion and communication, and sight (awareness and perception) and communication. Crystals which are blue in color are usually used for the throat chakra and can be harnessed to aid in all aspects relating to communication, truth, and wisdom.

Crystals for the Throat Chakra: Amazonite, Turquoise, Aquamarine, Blue Lace Agate, Blue Topaz, Lapis Lazuli, Chalcedony, and Sodalite.

The Third Eye Chakra

Introduction: THE BROW

Color: **Indigo** (mid-night blue)

Element: **Ether**

Indigo energy affects the pituitary gland that governs the hormones of the other endocrine glands. It is the conductor of the orchestra. Indigo is a great purifier, and calms and soothes the mind. It influences the organs of sight, smell and hearing. The third eye links us to our higher self, can broaden the mind and free our inhibitions. It also cleanses psychic currents, obsessions and phobias. Indigo is therefore a very powerful color vibration- the stones are cleansing, purifying, and mind expanding.

The third eye chakra is located between the brows. In Sanskrit, ajna translates as command, therefore, it is no surprise that this chakra is known as the command center. The third eye is responsible for all aspects relating to perception, sight, and psychic awareness. It links to the ability to perceive subtle energy, spiritual illumination, dream states, and wisdom and learning. If you have a strong third eye chakra you are highly intuitive and connected to your spiritual body. You are also aware of the interconnected, metaphysical nature of reality and may tend to be an idealist, committed to higher truths or vision in some way. Crystals which embody this energy can be connected to release any blockages, or detrimental beliefs or viewpoints holding you back. Crystals are usually purple, indigo, or violet in color, however, can also be white or clear/ opaque. The third eye chakra is the chakra which tends to become naturally activated when working with subtle energy and connecting to crystal energy fields, as it is the direct link to psychic phenomena and invisible (subtle) energy.

Crystals for the Third Eye Chakra: Lapis Lazuli, Sodalite, Labradorite, Azurite, Celestite, Sapphire, Fluorite, Clear Quartz, Moonstone, and Amethyst.

The Crown Chakra

Introduction: THE CROWN

Color: **Violet**

Element: **Ether**

The crown chakra links to the function of the brain and the pineal gland. Violet ray energy stimulates the hormone melatonin and also produces hormones that control other biological functions. We know that a deficiency of melatonin can result in the illness known as Seasonal Affective Disorder, or SAD, which results from lack of natural sunlight. The crown chakra is associated with the sympathetic nervous system, and imbalance of energy in this area leads to headaches, migraine, and other problems related to the head and scalp. Violet energy soothes the nervous and mental disorders, neurotics, and is useful in the treatment of tumors and concussion. The crown chakra also connects us to the spiritual world (this does not mean the realm of the dead but rather the greater part of our environment which vibrates at too high a frequency to be detected by our 5 senses, or by our present level of technology). This chakra can protect us from negative forces from other dimensions. Violet stones thus help our quest for spirituality, and help expand our mind on a path of enlightenment and self-development.

Finally, the crown chakra is the last of the 7 major chakras. It is essentially the embodiment of pure light and universal consciousness. The crown chakra symbolizes and relates to self-realization, enlightenment, white light, purity, transcendental awareness, compassion, and connection with the divine. It also represents 'coming home' due to its link to kundalini. Spirit is grounded into the human body through the kundalini and it achieves this through the harmony, unification, and free flow of energy through all the chakras. Universal symbols and associations of the crown chakra include Christ and Christ consciousness,

Buddha and enlightenment, Krishna consciousness, the diamond, masters and ascended masters, and spiritual guides. Crystals which can be used to connect to qualities associated with the crown chakra include white and gold.

Crystals for the Crown Chakra: Celestite, Selenite, Sapphire, Sugilite, Amethyst, Diamond, Pearl, and Clear Quartz.

Kundalini: Wholeness, Harmony and Balance

Pure white sunlight contains everything necessary to maintain life on earth. The electro-magnetic radiations flood down onto the earth and penetrate everything on this planet. Light energy penetrates into the earth, into the mountains and caves. The magnetic energy is absorbed into the earth and rocks, and crystals begin their growth in the darkness using this energy. When we

bring crystals out into the light, they reflect the colors of the rainbow. Crystals, as we have learned, are living entities containing the life force, which they hold and can release once awakened. The growth of a crystal, just like ours, is a long and continuous one. Indian gem therapists believe that the crystals are composed of the seven rays, which are primeval, formative forces in nature, and it is through the combination of these forces that tangible forms are produced. Gems are **pure light energy**, and the colors of gems reflect the color energy with which the particular gem is empowered. When white light passes through a gemstone, some color wavelengths are absorbed while other vibrations pass through. The color passing through the gem is amplified and the healing quality of the color can be used in crystal treatments.

The human body is designed so that it is self-building and self-healing. By combining our energies with that of gems, the self-healing processes can be stimulated. This only occurs when there is an energy balance between body, soul and mind. Crystal healing uses the crystals and the color energy they contain to stimulate the bodies energy system into activity and recharge it with energy. And you may have already begun to see the similarity and connection… Just as a multi-spectrum of color and light can be found in the crystal queen/ kingdom, we ourselves are made up of light. **Rainbow energy**- that is the colors of the rainbow- flows through us on a subtle level. This is where kundalini comes in.

Kundalini is our life force and it is the whole, balanced and holistically-integrated self. When there is a free flow of energy from root to crown and crown to root, so when there are no blocks or imbalances- and when there is a harmony and unity between the 7 major chakras- kundalini is activated. It is important to be aware of kundalini energy in relation to crystals and their healing powers and metaphysical properties, because, just like a quartz crystal and other unique crystals such as the diamond, your kundalini is the embodiment of **pure light**. Light and a connection with the divine flows through you when your kundalini is whole and balanced, and when there is harmony between your 7 major chakras.

Individual gemstones can be used to heal and remove distortions or imbalances from each individual chakra, yet a few rare gems can be used to energize, heal and balance your whole chakra system, therefore your kundalini. Again, kundalini is your **life force**- it is responsible for health, longevity and personal power and authority. When your kundalini is strong and your chakras balanced (and healthy) you are self-empowered, self-aware, and more spiritually connected. Your intuitive mind is also activated, you are in tune with your intuition and "gut feeling" or inner voice. Psychic gifts and abilities, and an increased sensuality also come about with an active kundalini. So, working with crystals either through meditation, frequent handling, using them in self-healing or wearing them as pendants, allows you to **raise your inner vibration** and activate your vibrant life force; so that greater states of health, awareness and vitality can shine through.

This brings us onto crystals and **color**. Remember that you are a rainbow, even if on the subtle and spiritual planes!

Crystals and Color

Just like chakras, colors can be used and explored to aid in crystal healing and shifting vibrations within. This is because every color emits its own frequency; they each have their own vibrational quality associated within. During a crystal's formation, light energy penetrates deep within the earth's structures. The electromagnetic energy which radiates down is essentially where a crystal begins its journey. Crystals start in the darkness and subsequently absorb the vibrational qualities of the light and magnetic energy being emitted. Crystals are therefore living entities with a life force.

We can look to the healing quality of the color associated to understand which crystals can be used for our benefit. We briefly explored this in 'The Chakra System', however, let's have a deeper look at the main colors and how they relate to the crystal queen and kingdom.

Red

Red crystals and gemstones are warming, energizing, and stimulating. They bring strength, connection to the earth and body, and have a grounding and stabilizing influence. The vibrational frequency of red can provide vitality and be used for issues related to the reproductive organs. You can also connect to red to accept responsibility, duties, and practical realities which you may be against.

Key qualities: energizing, stimulating, grounding and stabilizing.

Orange

Orange crystals are perfect for situations of shock, trauma, fear, or anxiety. This is due to the warming and comfort bringing effect. Orange crystals help bring greater feelings of connection, emotional warmth and intimacy, and can be used when dealing with any friendship, love, or family issues. They increase passion for life and a sense of joy. They can also be connected to if you are lacking in inspiration and need a creative or imaginative spark.

Key qualities: warming, comforting and encouraging.

Yellow

Yellow crystals have a stimulating and energizing effect. They generally increase confidence, clarity, and feelings of self-empowerment, and can help greatly with all aspects relating to the self. Ego, will, inspired action, life direction, and focus all can be enhanced with yellow gemstones. Yellow is also a very empowering color due to its connection to fire and the sun, therefore, in addition to energizing and stimulating they help calm anxiety, intense or difficult emotions, and nervous tension.

Key qualities: stimulating, energizing, inspiring and calming.

Green

Green gemstones are primarily for the heart. They have a balancing, calming, and warming effect, however, can also be stimulating due to their effect on personal growth and development. Some green crystals act as emotional stabilizers whilst others inspire people into heart-centered action. They can be used to aid in nature-orientated pursuits such as when working with herbs, flower essences, or essential oils. All qualities such as empathy, kindness, compassion, and caring can be enhanced with green gemstones.

Key qualities: warming, comforting, harmonizing and balancing.

Light Blue

Light blue gemstones aid in communication and bring feelings of peace and inner contentment. They have a gentle effect and therefore are usually used for problems relating to feelings and expressions. This color frequency also helps release emotions and tensions and generally brings a feeling of lightness. Blue crystals are cooling, soothing, and subtly motivating.

Key qualities: cooling, soothing, calming and stimulating.

Dark Blue

Dark blue gemstones bring depth and richness with a majestic-like feel. They can be used to enhance musical and creative pursuits which require you to connect with the higher mind, the divine, or metaphysical wisdom. For this reason, they can have a stimulating and energizing effect.

Key qualities: stimulating, energizing, and inspiring.

Purple and Indigo

Purple and indigo crystals are purifying, calming and soothing. They can influence, inspire, and expand the mind, and relate to the third eye, subtle perception, and psychic and intuitive sight. Indigo specifically is a very powerful color vibration and has links to ancient wisdom, esoteric knowledge, and the higher self. There is also a majestic quality to purple and indigo. Crystals with these colors make excellent meditation and self-contemplation stones, in addition to relating to spiritual enhancement.

Key qualities: cleansing, purifying, soothing and influencing.

Violet, White, and Clear

White and clear crystals bring clarity, purification, and harmony. They can be connected with to amplify life force energy and develop a freer flow of energy through the chakras. These colors can also be tuned in to clear blockages and bring harmonious flow to the kundalini. Violet, white, and clear crystals generally have a soothing and cleansing effect, and violet, in particular, can be stimulating on certain positive qualities such as sight and perception. Violet also has a stimulating effect on the pineal gland and nervous system.

Key qualities: purifying, harmonizing, clearing and soothing.

In Chapter 4, we explore specific crystals in detail.

Cleansing, Grounding, and Charging: The Importance of Clearing

One of the most significant things you will learn to do on your journey of connecting with crystals and integrating them into your life is to cleanse, clear, ground, charge, and set your intentions. As you are aware, crystals are conscious living entities. They hold unique vibrational and healing qualities and have been formed directly from the earth, the elements, and the light and astrological frequencies from space. As with any living thing, organisms can become polluted. Cleansing, therefore, is something you will grow to learn as highly significant, and if not, essential to your personal relationship with gemstones and receiving their energies.

In addition to cleansing, charging and grounding your crystals will make the energy and benefits so much more profound, as will intention setting. Let's look at these in detail.

Cleansing Crystals

Cleansing crystals is essential as all crystals pick up on energy. Now, before we take this at face value it is important to understand what this fully means. Crystals pick up on and absorb other people's energies. This means that all thoughts, intentions, projections and unseen elements become absorbed into the crystal's electromagnetic energy field. These 'unseen things' can be very detrimental as can thoughts and projections. Hidden and subconscious wounds, traumas, inner pains, hardships, life problems, and 'stuff' gravitate towards the crystal whose purpose is to heal and help through their energy, thus 'polluting' the crystal's energy field. Various stories, realities, traumas, pains, and things which need healing take up space- energetically- simultaneously weakening the crystals' purity and function to heal.

Not only are the real-life pains and daily struggles unconsciously projected harmful, but some people actually intentionally harm and weaken the crystals' healing effect. A lot of people don't understand crystals; therefore, they project unhelpful and destructive thoughts such as 'I don't believe,' 'you can't possibly heal,' and "people who believe in crystals are crazy.' These become absorbed into their energy field and- just like when someone is mean and hurtful to us- it affects them! Imagine someone standing there belittling, undermining, and projecting negative intentions and illusions towards you? So, in this respect, crystals can often become polluted and filled with healing energy weakening thoughts and intentions before they even reach us. This brings us on to the power of cleansing.

Cleansing is essentially washing away all impurities, ill thoughts, and negative vibrations in water. Water is representative of purity, the subconscious, and creation; it is the life giver. Our bodies consist of just over 70% water and the earth itself is mainly water, even though we call her planet earth (planet water or ether?). Cleansing crystals in water, therefore, allows for the crystal to be restored back to its original and unique vibration. Water brings a crystal back to ground zero, free from harmful and 'heavy' energies.

Cleansing is so simple yet so effective. It only needs to be done for as little as 30 seconds to 2 minutes for effect, however, it can also be done by leaving your crystals in a bowl of fresh cold water for as long as you intuitively feel right. Mountain, spring, purified, or filtered water works best. It is also important to set your intention, even if only briefly, for the healing and cleansing qualities of water to be enhanced. A simple blessing such as 'thank you water for cleansing this crystal' can work wonders.

Grounding

It is also important to ground your crystals after cleansing them. Technically speaking, this technique is not essential (unlike cleansing and charging), however, it can be highly useful. Grounding is essentially placing your crystal in the earth so it becomes merged with the earth's energies. This can be as simple as burying it under some soil in your garden or placing it next to a tree or special flower (such as a rosebush which links to the heart). This way, the earth's electromagnetic energy field interacts with the crystal's, acting as a form of re-charge.

It is important to note with grounding that not all crystals respond well. Gemstones specifically for intuitive, inspirational, and higher self-energy, for example, do not particularly benefit from grounding. This is due to their high vibrational frequency linking with the higher mind and spiritual realm, and the earth's energy is of course very grounding. Crystals which can be enhanced from grounding, therefore, include red, brown, and green crystals, and ones which naturally embody grounding qualities such as tree moss agate.

For higher mind, airy, and psychic and subtle energy-based crystals, you could always place them on top of a money tree, aloe vera or houseplant (as opposed to burying them in the earth!).

Charging

Like cleansing, charging your crystals will really allow you to receive the full effects of the healing qualities and benefits. There are two ways to charge a crystal. The first is through sunlight and the second through your hands and intention.

The sun is essentially a source, pure energy, and life force. Leaving a crystal in direct sunlight for as little as half an hour to an hour can, therefore, have a great effect. As everything is interconnected and we live in an energetic universe, the crystal absorbs the energies directly from the sun, enhancing the qualities of the crystal. For example, leaving an amethyst in sunlight for a few hours would amplify its energetic properties (intuition, enhanced dream abilities, and recall and connection to the higher self).

Charging your crystals in sunlight amplifies, energizes, and increases the metaphysical healing qualities they have been formed from.

In addition to sunlight, you can also charge your crystals in moonlight. Just as the sun's energy acts as a boost and amplifier, the moon's energy can do the same for crystals with qualities associated. There wouldn't be much use charging obsidian or carnelian in moonlight (as they both relate to non-lunar qualities as you will discover later), however, charging moonstone, quartz, or pearl in the moon's energy can have some profound effects.

Let's briefly explore some of the characteristics and energetic qualities of the sun and moon (sunlight and moonlight).

Charging Crystals through Your Hands and Intent (Crystal Programming)

The second method to charge your crystals is with your palm chakras- the chi which flows through your hands and every living thing- and your intention. Chi is a form of subtle energy which is known by some as the universal life force. Chi is essentially a metaphysical quality present in crystals, ourselves, and all life on earth. When we open ourselves up to subtle energy, raise our vibrations, and connect to the crystal world, we naturally become more open to chi. We also naturally are able to channel chi and healing energy more powerfully.

Charging crystals in this way is also known as programming, as you are literally programming the crystal with a specific quality, intention, or amplified energy.

To charge your crystal, begin by holding it in your left hand. Your hand should be flat with the palm facing upwards and the crystal directly in the center. Hold your right hand over the top a few centimeters away and close your eyes. Bring your awareness inside and be conscious of the physical and energetic sensations within and around your hands and the crystal.

Perform 8-10 deep breaths to fill yourself with chi and, once you feel calm inside with a connection to the crystal, speak some intentions gently into it. These intentions can be anything from the following:

'Thank you for your beautiful, healing and loving energy.'

'I bless you with love, light, wisdom, and healing.'

'Thank you, sun, thank you moon, thank you water, thank you air, thank you earth. I am open to receiving your healing energy.'

'I recognize your healing power and I open myself to receive whatever wishes to shine through.'

Or anything you intuitively feel works best. The key element to remember with charging and programming your crystal is that everything is consciousness. All life has a conscious energy field and through our thoughts, we can actively influence the energetic qualities of physical matter. In other words, our thoughts and intentions hold great power to activate the already present qualities and energetic healing frequencies of crystals.

Once you become more familiar with working with crystals and harnessing their powers you will begin to get more creative and confident in your ability to program crystals. You may naturally find yourself developing specific intentions for specific types of crystals, for example for gemstones relating to enhancing intuition, psychic abilities, or inspiration: 'I charge you with love, light, wisdom, and healing energy to shine through. I recognize your power and open myself up to your intuition, sight, and connection to the divine.'

Chapter 9: Choosing The Right Crystal

Being a newbie in the realm of crystal healing, one of the first lessons to learn is how to choose the right crystal for yourself and/or for the chosen purpose. The trick is this statement, 'You don't choose crystals. They choose you!'

Finding the Right Crystals in a Brick-and-Mortar Store Using Your Intuition

Walk into an established and well-reputed crystal store, and do nothing but look around initially. Walk around the store and identify if you feel any kind of emotional or visual attraction toward any particular crystal. The exercise takes a bit of time, and therefore, you must be patient with yourself. If you don't connect with any crystal for the first time, go back and return the next day.

Typically, if you are looking at a set of crystals, and you feel drawn toward one of them, then it is usually a vibrational match for your energy frequency. Take your eyes away from the stone that you feel an initial attraction for and, after some time, look at it again, and see how you feel.

Hover your dominant hand over the crystal or better still, hold it in your hand. Close your eyes and observe any subtle energy changes or vibrations you feel in your body. If you do, then this crystal is definitely calling for your needs. You can go ahead and choose it.

Remember that you may not always be able to discern the subtle vibrational changes in energy when you hold the crystal, especially as a beginner. In such cases, go ahead and make your choice based on your initial reaction. Use the crystal for a week or two, and observe your experiences. With patient practice, you will find it increasingly easy to discern energy changes regardless of how subtle they are.

So, regardless of what you want the crystal for, trust your gut instinct and play along with it. And one of the most valuable suggestions you can get is to not overthink excessively about your choice of crystals.

In fact, you don't need to study and research the different types of crystals available before making your choice. Choose what attracts you, and then do a bit of research. More often than not, you will see that your choice of crystal matches with your needs.

Another piece of useful advice you can use is to take things slowly. First, take one crystal, use it for a week, and see how you feel and connect with its auric energy. Observe and make notes of the behavioral and attitudinal changes in your life, in yourself as well as those of others around. The changes are likely to be very subtle, and, therefore, you must focus a little more than normal to observe.

Once you are fine with what is happening, then you can go back and choose more crystals for yourself.

Finding the Right Crystal in a Virtual Online Store Using Your Intuition

Nearly all virtual stores will have some basic information and pictures of the crystals for you to choose from. Look at one page of pictures, and see which one attracts you the most or on which of the crystals do your eyes linger.

Most often, the crystals you are attracted to in a particular situation is relevant in your life for that time. Instead of trying to find 'scientific and logical' reasons for your attraction, know and believe that your intuition is telling you what your soul needs. Which is why it is important to trust your intuitive powers and go along with its calling.

Until now, you are focusing on the crystals you are drawn to. You can shift your perspective for a moment, and focus on those crystals and gemstones that you feel repelled against. Those are the ones that you must definitely avoid choosing at that point in time because your intuition is telling you that the vibrational energy of that crystal is not aligned to your present needs.

Receiving a Crystal as a Gift

Sometimes, people can choose crystals for you, and when this happens, remember that the crystal has chosen to be with you even without you stepping out to make your choice. The stone has literally found a way into your life through a caring friend. If you receive a crystal as a gift, then accept it wholeheartedly with an open mind in the same way you accepted your initial attraction to stone when you went shopping for your own crystal.

However, receiving crystals as gifts usually comes at a later stage in your crystal collection journey. As you increasingly connect with crystals and through them to the universal power, your needs and desires are caught onto by the universe and using the law of attraction, the universe finds a way to get your crystals delivered to your doorstep. Typically, such deep desires to have a particular crystal to achieve a particular purpose are realized in the form of gifts.

Taking this point in the reverse direction, suppose you lose a crystal. Yes, you will feel bad about losing it, and you could shed a few tears and be disappointed in yourself for being careless and not looking after your beloved stone well. However, you must remember that it is very likely that the stone has served its purpose in your life, and the universe has found a way to pass on the benefits of its power to someone else that needs it. So, just like how crystals find their way to you when you need them, they could go away from you when their purpose is served. Therefore, learn to let go if you lose anything in your life.

Choosing a Crystal Based on Its Properties

If you are looking for a crystal for a particular ailment or problem, then you can find gemstones that are known to help in solving these problems. For example, there are specific crystals like aventurine that has vibrational energy suitable to boost confidence. So, if you are looking to build confidence, then you can choose an aventurine.

In fact, aventurine is not the only stone that helps to boost confidence. Even crystals like bloodstone, carnelian, etc. are great for this problem. You can go through all the crystals based on a specific property you are looking at, and then make your choice from among these using your intuition's guide.

Finding the Right Crystal Using the Pendulum Dowsing Method

Using the pendulum dowsing method is a bit of an advanced technique, and requires you to have a bit of experience. Yet, even for a beginner, it makes sense to know how it works. Use the following steps for this method:

Find the right dowsing pendulum - Think about what kind of dowsing pendulum you would like to have. There are numerous crystal-based pendulums you can choose from, and also you can make a simple one at home too. An easy-to-make do-it-yourself dowsing pendulum needs a tea bag or a favorite bead or a favorite crystal or stone tied to the end of a string.

Cleanse and clear the pendulum of negative energies - If you already have a pendulum that you use for your divination purpose, then you might already know how to cleanse and clear your instrument.

Connect with and build a lasting relationship with your pendulum - You have to learn the language of the pendulum and connect with it to build a lasting relationship with your divination instrument. This step is important so that you understand and catch the messages that your pendulum is trying to tell you every time you use it for divination purpose including choosing the right crystal. Follow these steps to connect with your pendulum:

• Take a few deep breaths and ground yourself

• Seek support and help from the universe to help you achieve your purpose. You can use your own prayers or ask in simple language for help.

• Ask some basic questions to your pendulum to understand yes, no, or maybe answers it might choose to give. For this to work, remember to ask questions to which you already know the answers. Other ways of setting up a communication channel with your pendulum include:

Ask your pendulum, 'what is a yes?' and wait for the answer. It could move clockwise or counterclockwise. Make a note of this reply.

Next, ask your pendulum, 'What is a no?' or 'What is maybe?' and wait for the answers, and make suitable notes.

• Another way you can establish a communication channel with your pendulum is by getting responses to questions like:

Am I male or female?
Is it right that I am [fill in your age] old?
Are my eyes brown?
Do I enjoy reading?

The yes/no answers given by your pendulum will help you know how your pendulum is connecting with you.

Now, your pendulum is ready for use. Place your chosen crystal on a table and hold your pendulum over it. Watch for the signs given by your divination instrument and make your choice of whether you want to take this crystal or not. Your divination pendulum is a great tool to help you make many choices.

Other Elements of the Crystal to Focus On

While being guided by your feelings and intuition is the best way to choose your crystals, here are some more elements you should focus on while making your choice:

Form of the crystal - Typically, most crystals emit their power through the edges, and the most intense power comes from their tips. The form of the crystal you choose depends on its use. A stone that has multiple edges and splintered tips will radiate and emit its energy through all the edges and tips. However, the energy radiation may not be uniform when you use these forms.

Spheres, on the other hand, radiate their energy uniformly. However, the radiation from a spherical-shaped crystal will be weaker than when emitted through an edge. Usually, crystals that are cut to a specific shape tend to have more radiation power while tumbled stones tend to radiate energy more gently, softly, and harmoniously than other forms.

Quality of the crystal - Stones that display the unique characteristics of a particular crystal are of better quality than those that don't display the expected traits. For example, the quality of clear quartz is determined by its brightness. The more cloudy it is, the lesser the quality of the clear quartz.

On the other hand, a transparent ruby is more powerful than an opaque one. And yet, you must remember that the looks and profile of stone are less important than its potential power. Follow your gut feeling here too, and even if you feel a stone is not what it appears, but your intuition powers are on a high when you hold it, then the crystal could be right for you. Remember that sometimes crystals simply need cleansing and cleaning to regain their original luster.

Size of the crystal - The larger the size of the crystal, the more power it can radiate. A small-sized amethyst will radiate power only to a short range of distance whereas a big druse or collection of amethyst crystals can radiate power to cover an entire room. Therefore, you must choose the size of your crystal based on your needs.

For example, if you want to place a stone so that it radiates its power to clear the negative energies from a big room, then you must choose a large-sized crystal or maybe even a cluster of crystals. However, if you want to wear a crystal around your neck, then you can choose a small one because the contact of the stone with your skin will enhance absorption by your body.

Most experienced crystal healers believe in gentle and slow healing rather than a blasting effect. Make your choices sensibly and prudently based on the above three factors.

Other Tips While Choosing Your Crystal

Here are some more tips you can use while choosing your crystal.

Avoid making your choice when you are feeling mentally or emotionally imbalanced - For example, if you are tired, stressed out, angry, or even excessively happy, don't go shopping for crystals. It is likely that wrong ideas find their way into your head based on the emotions you are experiencing.

Don't choose crystals for others - In fact, as a beginner, completely avoid choosing crystals and gemstones for other people, including your loved ones and close friends. Remember that choosing a crystal has to do with matching an individual's energy vibration with that of the gemstone.

You will not be able to read and decipher someone else's energy vibrations during the initial phases of crystal healing lessons. Even if someone gives you permission to choose crystals for them, it takes a lot of study and practice, and only the top scholars in the realm can confidently do this work accurately. It is best to keep crystal healing and choosing methods to make choices for yourself alone.

Approach this exercise with an open mind - If you have chosen to access the power of crystals, then it means you are ready to take the plunge without over-analyzing things excessively. If you are looking for 'scientific and logical' proof of every action and thought, you are unlikely to find success. In fact, these doubts will color your choice and you are bound to make mistakes. Therefore, it is imperative that you approach the exercise of choosing the right crystal with an open mind, and trust your intuition to guide you.

Finally, sometimes, despite your best efforts at trying to find a suitable crystal, you realize that you are not drawn to any of the stones that you have come across until now. You don't have to worry about it. Maybe, the time is not yet right for you to connect with the crystals that are shown to you by the universe through any channel.

If nothing attracts you powerfully, then accept the fact that the time is not yet right for you. Wait and keep your desires alive, and you will find your stone sooner rather than later. Another point of warning is to beware of buying crystals to simply hoard in your house. You run the risk of having stones with energy vibrations unsuitable and even harmful for your life.

Holding onto crystals without any purpose or meaning will reduce this exercise to a mere hobby, and crystal healing is more than a hobby. It is a calling. So, listen to your intuition and follow its guiding light. You will never be led astray by your own intuition. Believe in its power and take a leap forward.

And, of course, when you go on your crystal-finding journey, remember to expect the unexpected. You could go in search of finding lost love, and you could end up finding your true love, and realize that the love you lost had a greater purpose than you thought.

Chapter 10: What Is Crystal Healing?

A crystal is a solid rock that is arranged in a highly regular structure to give its specific shape. Each type of crystal has its own shape. Crystals are found naturally in nature. A process called crystallization can also make them manually. Crystals, however, can only form from a gas or liquid and, therefore, this is how they differ from stone and rock.There may be crystals within crystals, inclusions, shadows and light, and even other minerals growing inside of them.

Other than having different shapes, crystals also have different colors. The different colors are seen because of their specific geometry. The arrangement of the crystal lattice ensures that each crystal has a unique structure.

Crystals are used extensively in healing. They can be used in healing a wide variety of aches and diseases. Each crystal has its own unique energy. Crystals acquire their energy from their mineral content; different mineral contents is used for different healing purposes so one's choice of crystal is dependent upon the underlying problem

Crystal healing is considered a pseudoscience by some. Yet many use it as an alternate treatment to heal diseases and conditions. While there is no scientific proof for this technique, most who use crystal hearing will swear by this method. Crystal healing uses crystals to restore balance between the spiritual and physical parts of a person to heal them.

Practitioners or healers as they are called select crystals by their color and place them on parts of the body. Each crystal has a different type of property, and depending on what kind of healing is necessary, practitioners use different crystals.

There are various shapes of crystals and the list of crystals seems unending. However, they can be grouped based on their formation. Even though each crystal is different, they all have a similarity. Their shape is similar to each other but it is the minor changes that make each one unique.

Pointed crystals, tumble stones, shaped crystals, crystal clusters, and crystal chunks are the five groups of crystals that are used in healing.

Pointed Crystals have a pointy edge on one side and a flat edge on the other side. They are commonly used as a crystal wand during healing. They are used for cleansing and during meditation.

Tumble Stones are a mix of crystals. When various crystals join together, they form a tumble stone. They don't have a particular healing property.

Shaped Crystals are usually man-made. Since they are man-made, they are used depending on the type of cut they have.

Crystal Clusters, like the name suggests, are clusters of crystals. They help in balancing the atmosphere in an area and are used to help people cope with difficulties in life.

Crystal Chunks are similar to small grains and are mainly given to students to improve concentration.

Almandine Garnet
Unites the powers of strength and protection from both physical and psychic interference, bringing the wearer a sense of security and increasing the user's willpower and resistant to curses and negative energies. This stone is red/brown and enhances blood flow and aids in healing blood-related issues.

Andradite Garnet
Has deep connections to the earth with its deep hues of olive green, burnt yellow and is intrinsically connected to levels of higher of thinking, self-empowerment, and spiritualism. This type of Garnet represents safety and strength which brings it into association with the Heart, Earth, and Solar Plexus Chakras. Andradite is a great talisman for those feeling isolated or looking for love.

Grossular Garnet
Embodies the supportive and empowering energies flowing from mother earth and represents affluence, gratitude and service to others. This stunning incarnation of

Garnet comes in hues of golden yellow through to scarlet red and even bright and luscious shades of olive greens. This highly spiritual stone has connections to the Base/Earth Chakra, Heart Chakra, Solar Plexus and Sacral Chakras.

Pyrope Garnet

A truly enchanting gemstone sometimes referred to as 'living fire', a name which comes from its extraordinarily vivid colours of crimson scarlet to hues indigoes and violet. This stone influences both the Earth and Crown Chakras, bestowing on the user inspiration, enhanced creativity, vitality and warmth and consideration for others.

Spessartine Garnet

A magnificent stone exhibiting spellbindingly beautiful shades of dark gold, orange and light pale yellow hues when pure. This rare variety of Garnet is sometimes called the 'garnet of the sun' radiates energies that activate our inner critical thinking skills, and enhanced levels of analytically precise attention to detail, allowing the user to focus their attention with confidence and without fear. Its effect on our Sacral and Solar Plexus Chakras combine to strengthen willpower and boost creative tendencies.

Colour

Deep Red (Noble)

Red/Brown (Almandine)

Olive Green/Yellow (Andradite)

Red/Green

Crimson/Scarlet to Green (Pyrope)

Dark Gold/Orange Pale/Yellow (Spessartine)

Birthstone

January

February

May

October

Zodiac

Aquarius

Capricorn

Leo

Energetic Frequencies

Healing

Love

Luck

Prosperity

Chakras

The First Chakra or Base Chakra/Earth Chakra located at the bottom of the spine.

Hematite

Hematite has been in use since at least the time of the ancient Greeks, who used it in the production of rich blood red dyes. The natural Hematite (when polished) displays an iridescent, silvery sheen that is thought to mesmerise the beholder in the same way as moonlight on a clear night. Hematite is an essential addition to any healer's collection. It carries a high iron content thought to improve blood pressure, circulation, promote a healthy heart, and ease menstrual cramps. It is a stone that detoxifies body, aura, and the chakra network as a whole; it also absorbs toxins and pollution from the atmosphere around it, some examples of Hematite have been known to be so powerful that they carry a magnetic charge and it is thought that this quality aids in healing cuts and bruises, reduces stress and directly supports the overall healing process. When carried or worn Hematite brings clarity of thought, and boosts logic, memory, problem-solving skills, decision-making skills and focus. It strengthens determination and willpower, throwing off all self-imposed limiting beliefs giving way to freedom of expression, creativity, and ultimately the manifestation of one's will. Hematite is an extremely impressive 'grounding stone' that works by drawing negative energy and any emotional blockages affecting the aura or chakra network down to the Root Chakra where it is purged. Once the negative energy has been displaced Hematite's healing vibrations balance the entire chakra network, giving way to feelings of inner peace and joy.

Colour

Black

Grey

Zodiac

Aquarius

Aries

Energetic Frequencies

Love

Harmony

Healing

Peace

Chakras

The Root Chakra

Jade

Jade, otherwise known as the 'Dream stone' and holds deep connections to the spiritual world allowing a skilled gemstone user to acquire insights into ancient knowledge both occult and ritualistic (beware-this is not always a good thing). It is another stone that appears to us in a variety of colourful hues with many of them carrying their own individual associations, energies, healing properties and protective qualities but is traditionally assumed to be a green gemstone. Since ancient times it has been said that Jade blesses all that it touches with its energies of purity and serenity. Jade has a long history behind it and can be found in hundreds of legends as everything from talismans and amulets of luck to weapons, statues and even ceremonial burial suits. This gemstone, both ancient and noble has been prized for its medicinal purposes across Asia for thousands of years and since its influence has spread across the entire world. It was once thought that Jade ground to a fine powder and consumed in rice and water could heal ailments relating to the lungs, heart, kidney, spleen, vocal chords, bring balance to the body as a functioning system and prolonging the life of the user. Jade is sometimes called the Stone of The Heart and so holds strong connections to the Heart Chakra and influences the body's energetic network through the Heart Chakra, having a harmonising effect bringing clarity, balance, love and emotional clarity to the user. Jade is actually used to describe two kinds of minerals, with the difference in colourisation being due to the mineral composition of each stone, the two types of Jade are:

Jadeite is a sodium aluminium silicate which forms bright olive green, blue, black and even purplish hues.

Nephrite is comprised of calcium magnesium silicate which appears in hues of green, brown and white.

Black Jade

Black Jade boasts powerful energetic frequencies that are exceptional in their protective capabilities safeguarding the physical body and negating any unhelpful entities, negative energies, and the jealousy, anger, and fear projected by others. Black Jade is a stone that supports those working towards independence both at work and home by working to overcome any physical or environmental limitations and empowering the individual to take a stand against unfair situations, manipulative bosses, deceptions, and those who undermine others. In the home Black Jade inspires natural respect and equality within the household, its calming influence brings balance to an environment. As a healing stone Black Jade is known to fend off bacterial infections, protect against parasites and viruses, and give an overall boost to the body's healing process and pain threshold.

The Root or Base Chakra is linked to and opened by Black Jade which in turn invigorates the body and mind.

Blue Jade

Sometimes called 'The Stone of Serenity' Blue Jade is a Dianite crystal, a type of Jadeite carrying blues both dark and pale that can sometimes appear slightly greenish. Blue Jade connects us to the higher dimensions allowing access to usually hidden spiritual knowledge through its connection to the third eye and Crown Chakra and bringing peace and serenity for the user. Widely used by vibrational and sound healers for its calming effect on the body and synchronicity with the heart's natural rhythm. Blue Jade is a 'dream stone of wisdom' that alleviates feelings of excessive guilt, nagging doubt and feelings of depression through its supportive energy which activates both hemispheres of the brain keeping tempers well-balanced, enhancing decision-making skills and acting to release us from our self-imposed limits. Blue Jade's links to the

Throat Chakra carries powerful healing energies that soothe the vocal cords, heals joints, relieve the symptoms of inflammation arthritis and breathing conditions.

Colour

Green

Black

Blue

Birthstone

April

May

June

February

March

Zodiac

Taurus

Libra

Sagittarius

Energetic Frequencies

Magic

Protection

Chakras

The Heart or forth Chakra (green)

The Root or Base Chakra (black)

The Crown Chakra (blue)

Chapter 11: Steps To Make And Activate Your Own Crystal Grid

To amplify your crystal programming to healing and magic, there are many ways to construct a crystal grid as well as activate it.Crystal grids can be used to manifest your dreams and desires for money, healthy, happiness and power.

• Clean your sacred space using a powerful herb such as lavender or sage.

• Sit down and write your intentions on a piece of paper.

• Fold the paper with your intentions and place it in the center of your grid.

• Set up the rest of the crystals based on your intention, color and layout in an order towards the center.

•Inhale a deep breath and state your intention out loud.

• Keep a quartz crystal between you and the crystal grid.

• Visualize connecting the different crystals via the quartz crystal in a non-stop manner.

- Thank your crystals.
- You have activated your crystal grid!
- Leave it undisturbed for 40 days.

NB: Crystal grid layouts can be made based on the key colors of the crystals you want to power your intention or wish with.

Your First crystal kit

How to distinguish real from fake gemstone

No one wants to study geology in an effort to avoid being scammed with fake gemstones. Artificial glass and manufactured quartz are the latest craze to those that don't understand the power behind the source. However, there are a few signs to look for when purchasing crystals to know how to tell if a gemstone or crystal is fake.

Glass is easy to Spot

Quartz is seasoned and cooled for centuries and has a geometrically perfect molecular structure, as all crystals do. Glass is quickly cooled to produce fast results. Because of the lack of time for conditioning, glass will have tiny air bubbles that have not been allowed to arrange in a pattern. There is one exception; clear Enhydro quartz refers to crystal that has fluid, gas or carbon bubbles beneath the surface. These bubbles will appear to have motion while glass bubbles do not.

Colored Quartz or Citrine

Quartz, citrine and amethyst glass pieces are often dyed to increase the clarity of the color. While the vibrant fuchsia, deep blue agate and yellow hues are beautiful, they also point to being fakes. Look at the cracks and you will see a darkened color where the dye has gathered.

Unnatural formations

Tech companies use labs to manufacture high quality quartz crystals for electronics. Using a hydrothermal process, lower quality quartz can be forced into designed that promote new growth patterns. A stepped apex is the result and may form 3 facets instead of the usual 6 facet hexagon pattern. This process can also leave pieces with a greenish tint.

Hematite is not magnetic

Shops that advertise the power of hematite with magnetic characteristics are peddling man-made pieces. The power of the magnetism is due to the powdered iron oxide that is attached to a strong magnet. It is then buffed to a brilliant shine. Genuine hematite will not have magnetic properties.

Finding credible dealers can be a challenge when buying genuine crystals or gemstones. Price is not always a dead give-a-way, but the reputation of the company can put you on high alert. Do a little bit of research on new dealers and steer clear of inexpensive wares from China. Check out the credentials of website owners. There are many credible sources for finding real crystals and gems, but also some that only want to sell manufactured products.These are a few signs to know how to tell if a gemstone or crystal is fake.

How to choose your first crystal

Always choose crystals you are drawn to. Those are the ones you find pretty, sparkly, interesting and keep going back to. These will always help you, sometimes in strange and wonderful ways. It may be obvious to you when you check what they do why you were drawn to the specific crystal. They can also be predictive or they may be for someone close to you. Whatever their purpose, they will reveal it to you when needed. I've been drawn to specific quartz crystals, of which you can probably guess I have many, without knowing why. These will sometimes sit around for days, weeks, even on one occasion two years, but always there is a reason. Each is the right crystal for something or someone very specific. So when you're attracted to a specific crystal, don't worry about why. Trust yourself.

The most important thing when choosing a crystal is to trust yourself!

If it's a crystal for a specific purpose or gift for someone else then think about the reasons or person you are choosing the crystal for and be open to anything. Crystals will choose you; they'll appear to shout, sing, dance and jump off a shelf or almost leap out of your computer screen to get your attention.

Oh yes, I should have talked about crystals you "noticed", rather than ones you were "drawn to". It's those crystals that you don't like that will really help. You don't like them because they're touching something very uncomfortable and deep inside you, that you thought you'd locked away. (I've seen people burst into tears or be physically repulsed by a crystal!) Every now and then something starts to trigger it and you avoid the situation. You've avoided it for so long that you probably don't even know what it was in the first place. Now it's buried deep in your subconscious. And the crystals you don't like are going to bring it to the surface. When you work with these crystals you will probably feel emotional, perhaps have a good cry, get angry or anything else that lets the trapped emotion out for you. Sometimes it can be rough… but stay with it, it won't last long. And after that you'll feel better. So much better in fact that it will change your life! You will never have to avoid something again because of it (even if you didn't know what it was in the first place).

How to select crystal with a pendulum dowser

When you do, don't think about it too much. Simply stand in front of a selection of pendulums, or look at a page on this web site with a large selection, and select the first one you notice. What are you drawn to? What qualities do you want your pendulum to have? When you have your pendulum ask it if it's a good one for you! To do this simply identify your yes/no for yourself and ask if it is a good pendulum for you to work with. If it says yes fine, if not try another. Crystal pendulums are easier to work with when you start as crystals magnify energy making it easier for you to see a response. Hold the pendulum in your hand and ask a simple question to which you know the answer is "yes". Such as "am I a woman/man?" The pendulum will start to make a movement. Ask the opposite question and you should see a different movement. You have identified your "yes" and "no" and can now ask any question you wish. As with all spiritual tools pendulums respond to how they are treated. If you are serious your pendulum will always give you the correct answer (be aware of how you phrase your questions). If you treat it as a game or continually ask the same question over again it will respond accordingly! You can work with pendulum, dowsing rods or forked twig. A pendulum is more convenient, easier to transport and easier to work with over a client. Pendulums give you a physical external representation of your natural inner knowing. Once you have selected your pendulum, hold it over crystals one at a time and ask "do I need this crystal?" It's that simple.

Chapter 12: Popular Healing Crystals For Specific Physical, Emotional, Mental And Spiritual Needs

You now know how to use crystals for healing and how to select them based on your energy fields and chakras. The question now is which crystals should you use to address specific health conditions? This chapter will help you answer that.

The **calcite** is often recommended to individuals who wish to move on from a traumatic experience. Use the blue calcite if you are suffering from an abnormally rapid heartbeat. The most valuable characteristic of this crystal, however, is its ability to cleanse the chakras and unite the various dimensions of yourself (physical, mental, spiritual and emotional).

The **amethyst** is the crystal to turn to if you wish to achieve serenity. This is popularly used during meditation and when reformatting negative thinking patterns and increasing optimism. It's also popular among psychics because this crystal can strengthen intuitive powers. The amethyst cures emotional blocks. Additionally, you may use it to treat migraines and arthritic conditions.

An **agate** will help you release internal tension, be it emotional, spiritual or physical. If you wish to repair your wounded ego, then include a moss agate in your grid or carry the crystal with you. If you want to improve your disposition, then a snakeskin agate may prove to be useful. Meanwhile, the Botswana agate is the one you should use if you want to quit an addictive habit such as smoking.

The **aquamarine** is used to treat phobias. It offers stability of emotions and reduces psychological tension. If you're going through a tough emotional experience, draw strength from an **amazonite**. It is effective in relieving anxiety and strengthening your self-discipline. This crystal is also recommended to individuals with neurological disorders.

The **aventurine** is a cleansing crystal that is effective for the physical and the emotional body. When added to bathwater, it can help you relax and sleep better.

For individuals suffering from skin ailments, the **azurite** is the crystal of choice. It is also used to manage anxiety and prevent anxiety-related internal organ diseases.

The **beryl** is known to aid in treating glandular inflammation, eye diseases and colorectal cancer. If you feel that you are lacking compassion, then use an **apatite** to activate your heart chakra.

The **chrysocolla** has long been used by pregnant women to ease labor. It is also used to cure problems related with the female reproductive organs.

The **bloodstone** has the power to enhance one's circulation. Moreover, it cleanses the bloodstream.

If you're suffering from depression, you should own a **chalcedony**.This crystal is also used in treating leukemia and gallstones. **Chrysolite**, on the other hand, is used in battling infections caused by viruses.

For patients undergoing organ transplant, the **diopsite and enstatiate** help in preventing organ rejection.

For gout, use **chrysoprase**. This crystal can also enhance reproductive health for both males and females.

The **citrine** is a powerful crystal known to bring success to its bearer. Use it to attract abundance and enhance your self-confidence. Business owners may carry the crystal in their pockets when undergoing important transactions. Likewise, if you want to improve your finances, keep a citrine inside your wallet. Furthermore, this stone is believed to aid in improving the health of vital organs like the heart, the liver and the kidneys. This crystal is also recommended to those who are prone to causing self-harm.

The **diamond** is believed to aid in curing diseases of the pineal and pituitary glands. It is also powerful in getting rid of poisonous substances from the body.

For individuals who have been hurt in the past, the **emerald** can help them become more receptive to the idea of loving again.

Furthermore, this crystal is known for its usefulness in treating psychological disorders.

If you find yourself suffering from lethargy, invest in a **carnelian**. This is also useful in releasing oneself from the clutches of envy. Additionally, these crystals enhance creativity and sensuality. What's more, these stones are helpful in recovering your experiences from your past life.

If you need help in improving your concentration, then invest in a **fluorite**. It is also believed to be useful in treating diseases affecting the bones.

With its wide range of uses, the **garnet** has surely earned its name as the "Stone of Health". It is recommended for people suffering from hormonal imbalances. It can also prevent hemorrhage.

The **hematite** is known as the "Stress-fighting Stone". When someone sends negative energy towards you, wearing this crystal will cause that energy to return to the sender. It also has a purifying effect on the blood.

The **jade** is the stone to keep if you feel that you need to develop more ambition in life. Additionally, you can use it to cure thyroid and parathyroid diseases as well as illnesses involving the body's most vital organs.

The yellow **jasper** is used to boost the endocrine system, but its more valuable feature is its ability to align your etheric body. The red jasper can also fight infections affecting the digestive tract.

The **labradorite** clears and protects the aura and patches up energy leaks.

The **obsidian** is a protective crystal, which can save you from being mistreated by people with malign intentions.

The **lapis lazuli** may prove to be valuable if you're having trouble accepting yourself.

The **Malachite** balances your right and your left brain. Use it for better eyesight. As previously mentioned, those who want to recover from a failed relationship may use this crystal in conjunction with rose quartz. Additionally, it shields the bearer from radiation.

It's difficult to control negative thoughts and emotions towards others, but a **hemimorphite** can help with that.

The **moonstone** nurtures you emotionally. It promotes inner growth and at the same time, cultivates your psychic potentials.

If you're too high-spirited for your own good, the **onyx** will help in reining in your passions. Use it when deciding on a matter, which requires you to remain objective yet optimistic. This crystal is also recommended for those who want to have healthy skin. As you already know, this crystal is useful in releasing stress and negative energy buildup.

The **kunzite** helps in recovering from alcoholism. It is also recommended for individuals suffering from schizophrenia.

For people suffering from hematologic disorders, the cherry **opal** can be of help. The dark opal promotes healthy bone marrow. Meanwhile, the jelly opal improves your body's ability to retain the nutrients it needs.

The **pearl** is useful if you're having trouble commanding your heart. It is also recommended for people who are experiencing gastro-intestinal disorders.

The **morganite** ensures that the parasympathetic nervous system functions properly.

Wounded feelings heal more quickly with the aid of a **peridot**. This crystal also increases your physical strength.

Apart from healing the throat chakra, the **turquoise** is also useful in preventing you from being sidetracked from your most important goals. Additionally, this crystal is believed to possess age-defying properties.

The **pyrite** is useful in purifying the upper respiratory tract and improving digestion.

The **clear quartz** is quite possibly the most popular crystal among healers because of its unique ability to transform negative energy to positive energy. When you wear it on your body, it will effectively fend off radiation. If you have trouble coming up with creative ideas, take a few moments to gaze at the crystal.

The **rose quartz**, often called the "Love Stone", heals the heart chakra. If you find yourself in need of comfort, lay the crystal on the center of your chest for fifteen minutes.

The **topaz** helps increase appetite. It also promotes faster healing by enhancing tissue renewal. This crystal is recommended for people suffering from tuberculosis.

The **ruby** activates the heart chakra to help you become ready to receive love. More importantly, it enables you to find the balance between your emotional desires and your spiritual goals.

Apart from their beauty, the **sapphire**'s great characteristic is its ability to help the carrier achieve spiritual enlightenment.

The green **unakite** is effective in grounding. Disappointments have a way of making life seem out of focus, but this crystal will aid you in recovering from frustrations.

If you're really open to exploring your psychic powers, then the **sugalite** will help you develop visions. More than that, it will shield you from negative vibrations.

Use the **tiger's eye** if you want to develop more focus and become more responsible.

The black **tourmaline** is helpful in counterbalancing distorted energies. It is recommended for individuals suffering from dyslexia. The watermelon tourmaline is another heart chakra healer. It will help you feel more secure.

The **sardonyx** is recommended for those who are dealing with loss and grief.

The **sodalite** helps in activating your inborn psychic abilities. Use this crystal to make your mind more receptive to the inner sight. It also helps mute out mental clamor.

Chapter 13: How To Clean Your Crystal

Crystals are sensitive blessings of nature. They require cleaning – otherwise referred to as recharging – in order to ensure they can provide a consistent energy supply. The positivity of a crystals increases when you clean it the immediately after use. It is also recommended that you clean your crystal before using it for the first time. The cleansing process can be carried out at any time and any place. By cleansing your crystal you eradicate all types of unwanted energies from it. The negative vibrations that the crystal absorbs from its surrounding environment can negatively affect its healing power.

Physical Cleaning

Practice the following steps for proper physical cleansing of your crystal:

Dust it with a brush. Use light strokes to prevent damage to the sensitive stone. For brittle crystals, use a warm water bath and a toothbrush. Some people use dishwashing detergent and a scrubbing brush to remove dust particles.

For a muddy crystal, use oxalic acid. Add one parts oxalic acid to two parts water.You can also clean it using warm water with water pressure directed towards the mud. A wooden stick can be used to pick at the mud, but avoid using steel.

Cleansing Unwanted Vibrations

After a physical cleanse, negative energies and unwanted vibrations need to be removed from the crystal. The crystal powers reach the individual by passing through several sources and it absorbs all surrounding energies indiscriminately. You can use a proper salt burial ceremony for your crystal or bath your crystal in a salt water bath. Soak the crystal for at least seven hours to remove the negative energies and vibrations.

For stones used daily, you do not need to carry out daily salt baths. Instead the bath can be scheduled every two weeks. The water for the salt bath can be room temperature. If you have access to genuine sea water then that is best option. Otherwise a tablespoon of salt dissolved in the water will work as well

For crystals that cannot be soaked in salt water, you can choose to "smudge" it with sage or sweet grass. This process should last between three and seven minutes.

How to Charge and Activate Your Crystal

It is entirely your choice as to how to charge, or activate, your crystal. Place your crystal in a pouch or on a small cushion of soft material. Silk is a good option. Charging your crystal can be carried out according to the type of energy it requires, choosing from the following:

Solar Energy

Place your crystal outside in the sun for a few hours. The energy from sun can be amplified by covering your crystal with a clear glass, filled with clean water for optimal amplification.

Lunar Energy

This energy is related to inner fulfillment and magic. Put the crystal outside on a full moon for several hours. For aiding in illness place the crystal outside during a waning moon. For new beginnings, use the lunar energy from a waxing moon.

Earth Energy

This energy eliminates negativity and amplifies attraction and strength. Bury the crystal for few hours in the yard to absorb the earth energies. A soil pot is a good alternative if you do not have a yard.

Power Charge

Power charging the crystal helps to strengthen the stone and eliminate stubborn energies. To utilize this energy, place your crystal outside during stormy. Lightning is a must for the crystal to absorb negative ions.

Fire Energy

This energy purifies and cleanses the crystal. Simply pass the stone through the candle flame briefly.

Air Energy

If you are looking for improved communication and intellect, simply hold your crystal in presence of burning smoke. Sage is an excellent choice for this.

Chapter 14: Garnet

Garnet is a balancer stone usually found in Africa but also in the United States and Russia, this deep red gemstone has long been a symbol of compassion, love, purity, and truth-giving way to greater levels of spiritual awareness. Garnet exists in a number of forms including the brown/red Almandine (a Stone of Tangible of Truth), Merelini Mint Garnet, and Carbuncle, with the most prized being Noble or Precious Garnet. This highly revered gemstone is known to strengthen the wearer's ability to manifest into being realistic and positive realities within the psychical world around us. Garnet's connection to universal energies and mathematics creates a rational and calming atmosphere free from worry, panic and fear making it a great talisman for anyone branching out into new fields of study. Garnet is known as a stone for success, it has been said that if your business needs a boost place 3 Garnets on your desk and any business problems will find themselves resolved.

Garnet has been in use for 5000 years and Native Americans viewed the stone as sacred and one of the 12 stones making up the breastplate of the high priest due to its fast acting ability to expand one's awareness, light one's internal fires and enable the user to bring creative visions to reality. It is said that the power concealed within the Garnet is fuelled by an ancient bolt of lightning contained inside. Garnet is thought of as holding numerous medicinal uses including the stimulation and regulation of metabolism, the reduction of bodily toxins, the purification of blood and also in the cellular regeneration of organs like the heart and lungs and is even thought to bring answers to life's problems to wearers in their dreams. Many of the different types of Garnet have their own individual associations, energies and corresponding powers and protective qualities:

Conclusion

I hope this book was able to help you to understand and get to know this alternative way of healing better. Often times, alternative medicine and healing procedures are neglected by the medical community mainly because most of these products and therapies lack the necessary scientific and medical proof that most synthetic drugs have. They also usually laughed at because most scientists and medical practitioners call them as pseudoscience. They say that these alternative means of healing do not have enough scientific proof and basis, therefore they are inferior to the commercial and synthetic drugs that pharmaceuticals produce.

However, what most people don't realize is that these alternative medicines and therapeutic procedures, such as crystal healing, totally safe and natural ways of healing that are effective in making our health problems go away in just an affordable amount. You really have nothing to lose if you consider trying these alternative healing cures for your health problems. Just remember to always research first and now as much as you can about these alternative medicine because knowledge is power, always, and knowing something ahead of time can sometimes spell the difference between life and death.

I also hope that through reading this book, you were able to understand the basic concepts and techniques used in the art of healing through therapeutic crystals. I hope that you were able to grasp the essence of this alternative healing therapy and legitimately understood what it can really do for you and for others. The steps and techniques that were taught in this book were practically very easy to follow and try. Hopefully, you also learned by heart the different kinds of crystals, the different groups that they belong to and when to appropriately use the crystals in each color group in order to heal different kinds of illnesses.I also look forward to the fulfillment of my expectation that you were able to comprehend the concept of chakras and their importance.

I hope you were encouraged to practice, try and learn more about the art of crystal healing and use the knowledge that you were able to acquire from this book as a stepping stone into making yourself a certified crystal healer and an expert in this craft.

The next step upon successful completion of this book is to of course practice and apply what you have learned. Practice and application always go hand in hand in retaining the information that one has learned. Without practice, the skills that you learned from this book will never be enhanced and be cultivated. Try to quiz yourself if you really know the uses of the different crystals. Try to match the sickness with the appropriate crystals that can cure them. Try to find the location of your chakra without looking at a guide. Try the simple and different ways of cleansing your crystals. Try and try and practice until you have mastered the craft of crystal healing because that will be the only true way in succeeding.

May you also pass on to others the techniques and the knowledge about the art of crystal healing that you have learned in this book so that you can inspire others to learn and appreciate this kind of alternative therapy as much as this book has encouraged and inspired you to look into this bizarre but surely interesting therapeutic procedure. Remember as well to always learn and learn no matter how knowledgeable you become in crystal healing for there will always be new and available information, waiting for you to discover. A great crystal healer will never stop from researching and learning all about his or her craft.

Thank you and good luck!

www.ingramcontent.com/pod-product-compliance
Lightning Source LLC
Chambersburg PA
CBHW071824080526
44589CB00012B/911